THRIVING WITH EHLERS-DANLOS SYNDROME

A Guide to Living Your Best Life

BROOKLYN LUCAS

All rights reserved. No part of this book may be copied, shared, or transmitted in any way, whether by photocopying, recording, or other electronic or mechanical means, without the publisher's prior written consent. This excludes brief quotations used in critical reviews and certain other noncommercial uses allowed by copyright law.

This book is designed for educational and informational purposes only. The content aims to enhance understanding and appreciation of health-related topics. Any references to specific events, names, or copyrighted materials are included for commentary, criticism, or review.

The author and publisher are not responsible for any negative effects that may arise, directly or indirectly, from the information provided in this book.

TABLE OF CONTENTS

INTRODUCTION

Living with a chronic illness like Ehlers-Danlos Syndrome (EDS) is a journey filled with unexpected challenges, profound resilience, and a constant battle for normalcy. This book is an exploration of that journey through the eyes of Bella, a remarkable woman whose life story is both inspiring and heart-wrenching.

EDS is a group of genetic disorders that affect connective tissues, causing hypermobility, joint pain, and a myriad of other symptoms that can severely impact daily life. Bella's experiences provide a deeply personal look at the realities of living with this condition, offering readers a window into her world of strength, vulnerability, and hope.

When Bella first noticed the constant ache in her joints, she brushed it off as a byproduct of an active lifestyle. She had always been a dancer, her body moving fluidly through every performance, but now, even simple movements brought pain. The mornings grew harder, waking up to stiff limbs and a creeping sense of dread for the day ahead. Doctors' visits became a routine, each one more discouraging than the last, as vague diagnoses and ineffective treatments piled up. It wasn't until she found a specialist who recognized the telltale signs of Ehlers-Danlos Syndrome that she finally had a name for her suffering.

The diagnosis was both a relief and a curse. Relief, because Bella could finally make sense of the myriad symptoms that plagued her; a curse, because EDS had no cure. The reality of living with a chronic condition settled heavily on her shoulders. She cried for the life she thought she would have and feared for the future she couldn't predict.

Bella's days were a testament to quiet bravery. Each morning, she carefully planned her movements to conserve energy and minimize pain. Simple tasks like getting dressed or making breakfast became small victories. She learned to listen to her body, to rest when needed, and to find solace in the things she could still enjoy. Yet, the isolation of chronic pain was a constant companion. Friends didn't always understand why she canceled plans at the last minute, and even her family struggled to grasp the invisible nature of her illness.

Support came from unexpected places. Online communities of others with EDS offered camaraderie and understanding that she couldn't find elsewhere. Her mother, who initially seemed overwhelmed, became her fiercest advocate, researching tirelessly and accompanying her to every appointment. Bella's dance instructor adapted routines so she could continue to do what she loved without exacerbating her symptoms.

Through trial and error, Bella developed a toolbox of coping mechanisms. Physical therapy helped manage her pain, while meditation and mindfulness provided mental relief. She discovered a passion for painting, a creative outlet that allowed her to express emotions words couldn't capture. There were days when despair threatened to engulf her, but Bella's resilience shone through. She found strength in her vulnerability, allowing herself to grieve on the hard days and celebrating the good ones with unrestrained joy.

Bella's journey with EDS led her to advocacy. Sharing her story became a mission to raise awareness and support others facing similar battles. She spoke at events, wrote articles, and became a beacon of hope for many in the EDS community. Her advocacy work was a way to reclaim her narrative, transforming her pain into a source of empowerment.

Looking ahead, Bella remains cautiously optimistic. The future is uncertain, but her resolve is unwavering. She dreams of a world where EDS is better understood, where those with chronic illnesses are met with empathy and support. Bella's story is a testament to the human spirit's ability to endure, adapt, and find beauty even in the most challenging circumstances. Through her journey, she teaches us that while we cannot always choose the battles we face, we can choose how we face them, with grace, courage, and hope.

EHLERS-DANLOS SYNDROME

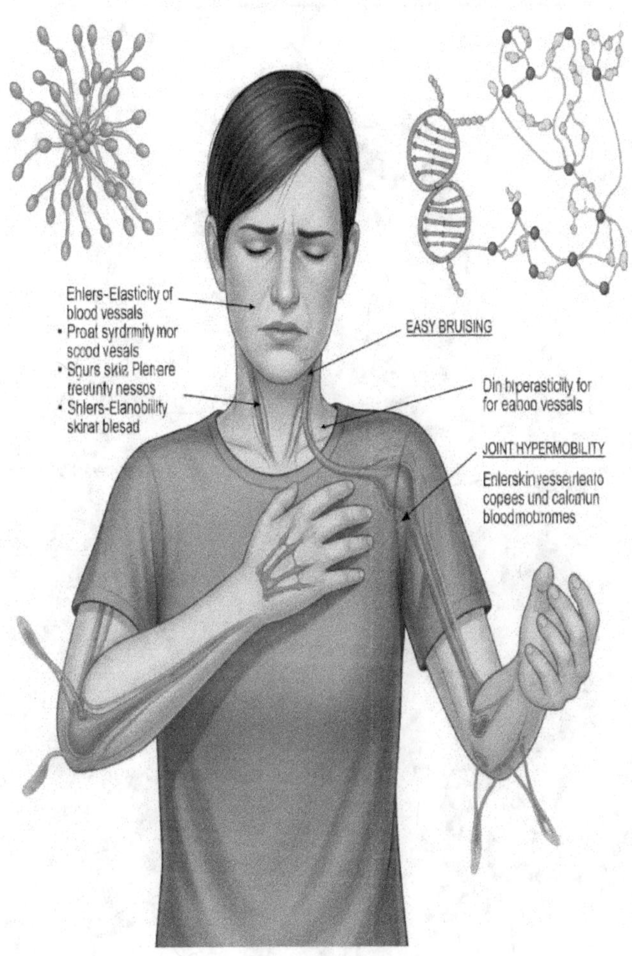

EHLERS-DANLOS SYNDROME

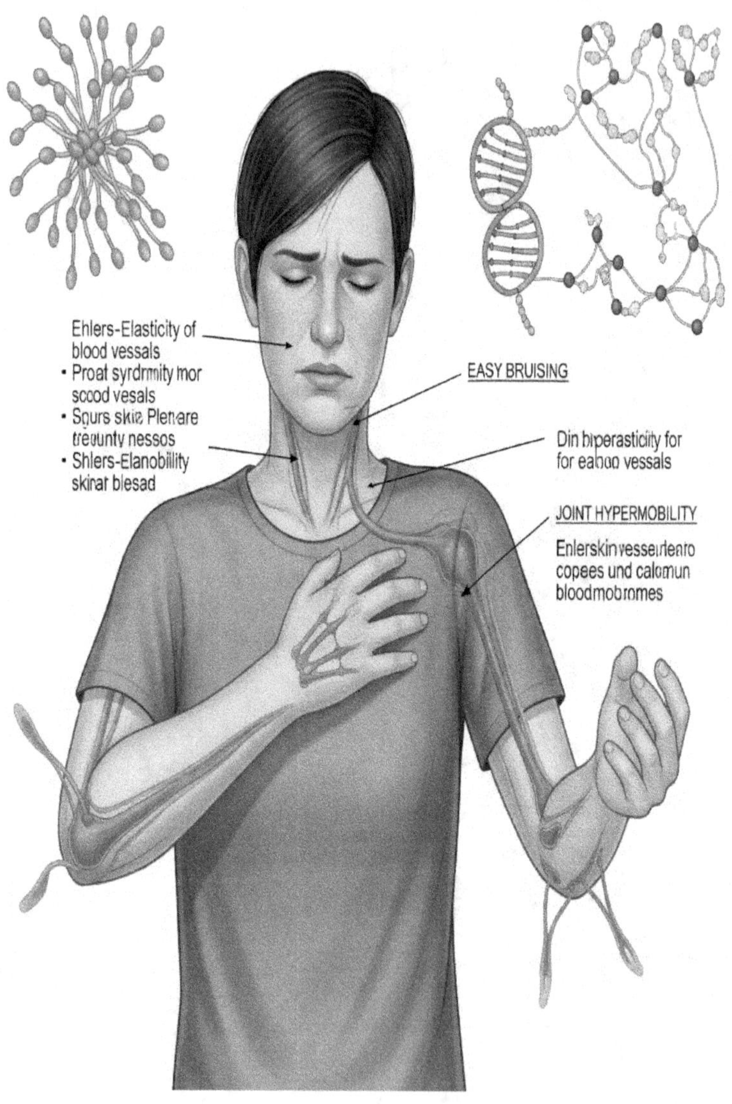

CHAPTER ONE

UNDERSTANDING EHLERS-DANLOS SYNDROME

1.1 What is Ehlers-Danlos Syndrome?

Ehlers-Danlos Syndrome (EDS) is a group of connective tissue disorders that can affect various parts of the body, including the skin, joints, and blood vessels. The connective tissues provide strength and elasticity to structures throughout the body, and when these tissues are defective, it can lead to the wide range of symptoms seen in EDS.

EDS is primarily known for causing hypermobility of the joints, skin that can be unusually stretchy or fragile, and a propensity for bruising. These symptoms occur because the body's connective tissues lack the normal strength and flexibility. The syndrome can be mild for some, but for others, it can lead to severe and life-threatening complications. Understanding EDS is the first step toward managing it effectively.

Connective tissues are made up of a complex mixture of proteins and other substances. One of the primary proteins involved is collagen, which acts like the glue that holds tissues together. In people with EDS, genetic mutations affect the production or structure of collagen, leading to the symptoms associated with the disorder. This genetic basis is why EDS often runs in families, though spontaneous mutations can also occur.

Awareness and understanding of EDS have increased over recent years, but it remains underdiagnosed, partly because its symptoms overlap with many other conditions. Comprehensive knowledge about EDS is essential for patients, families, and healthcare providers to ensure timely and accurate diagnosis and management.

1.2 The Different Types of EDS and Their Variations

Ehlers-Danlos Syndrome is not a single disorder but a collection of 13 distinct subtypes, each with its own set of characteristics and genetic causes. These subtypes vary widely in their symptoms and severity, making EDS a highly variable condition.

Hypermobile EDS (hEDS): The most common subtype, characterized by joint hypermobility, chronic pain, and frequent dislocations. The genetic cause of hEDS is still unknown, and diagnosis is typically based on clinical evaluation and family history.

Classical EDS (cEDS): Marked by highly elastic, velvety skin that bruises easily, and widespread atrophic scarring. Mutations in the COL5A1 or COL5A2 genes are usually responsible for this type.

Vascular EDS (vEDS): One of the more severe forms, vEDS is associated with a high risk of arterial, intestinal, and uterine ruptures. It is caused by mutations in the COL3A1 gene and requires careful management to avoid life-threatening complications.

Kyphoscoliotic EDS (kEDS): This type includes severe muscle hypotonia at birth, progressive scoliosis, and fragile eyes that are prone to rupture. It is often caused by mutations in the PLOD1 or FKBP14 genes.

Arthrochalasia EDS (aEDS): Characterized by congenital hip dislocation, severe joint hypermobility, and skin hyperextensibility. Mutations in the COL1A1 or COL1A2 genes are responsible for this type.

Dermatosparaxis EDS (dEDS): Known for extreme skin fragility, sagging, and easy bruising, this type is due to mutations in the ADAMTS2 gene.

Classical-like EDS (clEDS): Similar to classical EDS but without atrophic scarring, caused by mutations in the TNXB gene.

Brittle Cornea Syndrome (BCS): Involves thin, fragile corneas leading to a risk of rupture, alongside skeletal abnormalities. It is linked to mutations in the ZNF469 or PRDM5 genes.

Spondylodysplastic EDS (spEDS): Characterized by short stature, muscle hypotonia, and bowing of limbs, due to mutations in the B4GALT7, B3GALT6, or SLC39A13 genes.

Musculocontractural EDS (mcEDS): Features severe skin involvement and joint contractures, with mutations in the CHST14 or DSE genes.

Myopathic EDS (mEDS): Involves muscle weakness and joint hypermobility, caused by mutations in the COL12A1 gene.

Periodontal EDS (pEDS): Notable for severe periodontitis at a young age, along with other connective tissue problems. Mutations in the C1R or C1S genes are responsible.

Cardiac-valvular EDS (cvEDS): Characterized by severe cardiac-valvular problems alongside joint and skin symptoms, caused by mutations in the COL1A2 gene.

Each subtype of EDS presents unique challenges and requires specific management strategies. Understanding the specific type of EDS a patient has is crucial for effective treatment and improving quality of life.

1.3 Getting Diagnosed: A Patient's Journey

The journey to an EDS diagnosis can be long and fraught with frustration. Due to the wide range of symptoms and their overlap with other conditions, many patients see multiple specialists and receive various misdiagnoses before EDS is correctly identified.

Initial Symptoms and Seeking Help: For many, the path to diagnosis begins with recognizing unusual symptoms, such as frequent joint dislocations, chronic pain, or skin that bruises easily. These symptoms often lead patients to seek help from primary care physicians or specialists like rheumatologists or dermatologists.

Referral to Specialists: Due to the complexity of EDS, patients are often referred to geneticists or specialized clinics that can perform comprehensive evaluations. This stage may involve detailed family histories, physical examinations, and genetic testing.

Genetic Testing and Confirmation: Genetic testing plays a crucial role in diagnosing most types of EDS, particularly those with known genetic markers. For types like hypermobile EDS, where no specific genetic test is available, diagnosis relies heavily on clinical criteria and family history.

Emotional Impact and Support: Receiving an EDS diagnosis can be overwhelming. Patients may experience a mix of relief at finally having an explanation for their symptoms and anxiety about what the future holds. Support from healthcare providers, mental health professionals, and patient communities is vital during this time.

Creating a Management Plan: Once diagnosed, the next step is developing a personalized management plan. This plan may include regular monitoring of symptoms, physical therapy, pain management strategies, dietary recommendations, and lifestyle adjustments to protect joints and improve overall health.

Ongoing Care and Monitoring: Living with EDS requires continuous care and adaptation. Regular follow-ups with healthcare providers help manage symptoms and monitor for potential complications. Patients often become active participants in their care, learning to advocate for themselves and make informed decisions about their health.

Getting diagnosed with EDS is not the end of the journey, but rather the beginning of a new chapter.

With the right knowledge, support, and management strategies, individuals with EDS can lead fulfilling and empowered lives.

CHAPTER TWO

UNVEILING THE MYSTERY: THE SCIENCE BEHIND EDS

2.1 The Connective Tissue Conundrum: Understanding the Underlying Cause

At the heart of Ehlers-Danlos Syndrome (EDS) lies a fundamental problem with connective tissue, the material that supports, binds, or separates different types of tissues and organs in the body. Understanding this issue is crucial to comprehending the wide-ranging effects of EDS.

Connective tissues are composed of a complex network of proteins and other molecules that provide structure and strength to various body parts. One of the key components of this network is collagen, a protein that acts like a scaffold, giving tissues their tensile strength and elasticity. In people with EDS, genetic mutations disrupt the production, structure, or processing of collagen, leading to defective connective tissues.

The genetic mutations responsible for EDS can affect different types of collagen or other proteins that interact with collagen. For instance, mutations in the COL5A1 or COL5A2 genes affect type V collagen and are linked to Classical EDS (cEDS). Mutations in the COL3A1 gene impact type III collagen, leading to Vascular EDS (vEDS), one of the more severe forms of the disorder. Each type of EDS involves distinct genetic variations that result in specific symptoms and complications.

The process of collagen synthesis and assembly is intricate and involves multiple steps, from the initial production of collagen molecules to their assembly into robust fibers that can withstand mechanical stress. In EDS, mutations can occur at any stage of this process, leading to weakened or unstable collagen fibers. This instability manifests as the characteristic symptoms of EDS, such as hypermobile joints, fragile skin, and a propensity for bruising.

Moreover, the mutations in EDS are often inherited in an autosomal dominant manner, meaning only one copy of the defective gene from either parent is sufficient to cause the disorder. However, some forms of EDS are inherited in an autosomal recessive manner, requiring two copies of the defective gene (one from each parent) to manifest the condition. In some cases, these mutations can arise spontaneously, without any family history of the disorder.

The impact of defective connective tissue in EDS is systemic, affecting not only the skin and joints but also internal organs and blood vessels. This widespread involvement explains the diverse and often severe manifestations of EDS. Understanding the genetic and molecular basis of EDS is crucial for developing targeted therapies and management strategies that can improve the quality of life for those affected by this condition.

2.2 The Spectrum of Symptoms: How EDS Manifests in the Body

Ehlers-Danlos Syndrome (EDS) presents with a wide array of symptoms, reflecting the diverse roles that connective tissue plays throughout the body. These symptoms can range from mild to severe and can vary significantly among individuals, even within the same subtype of EDS.

1. Joint Hypermobility and Instability:

One of the hallmark features of EDS is joint hypermobility, where joints can move beyond the normal range of motion. This hypermobility often leads to joint instability, frequent dislocations, and subluxations (partial dislocations). These joint issues can cause chronic pain, early-onset osteoarthritis, and significant functional impairment. Activities that involve repetitive joint use or high impact can exacerbate these problems.

2. Skin Manifestations:

The skin in individuals with EDS is often remarkably elastic, soft, and velvety. It can be easily stretched and may return to its normal state slowly. Fragile skin that bruises easily and heals poorly is another common symptom, leading to atrophic scars that are thin and stretched. In some types of EDS, such as Classical EDS (cEDS), the skin is not only hyperelastic but also prone to splitting with minimal trauma.

3. Vascular Complications:

In Vascular EDS (vEDS), the most severe subtype, the walls of blood vessels and organs are particularly fragile. This can lead to life-threatening complications such as arterial rupture, intestinal perforation, and uterine rupture during pregnancy. These vascular issues require careful monitoring and immediate medical attention when they arise.

4. Musculoskeletal Problems:

Muscle weakness and hypotonia (reduced muscle tone) are common in many forms of EDS. These musculoskeletal issues can contribute to the overall instability of joints and complicate movement and physical activities. Scoliosis (curvature of the spine) and other skeletal abnormalities, such as kyphosis (outward spinal curvature), can also occur.

5. Gastrointestinal Issues:

Many individuals with EDS experience gastrointestinal problems, including chronic constipation, irritable bowel syndrome (IBS), and gastroesophageal reflux disease (GERD). These issues can result from the weakened connective tissue in the gastrointestinal tract, affecting its structure and function.

6. Cardiovascular Symptoms:

Apart from vascular complications, EDS can involve other cardiovascular symptoms like mitral valve prolapse and aortic root dilation. These conditions require regular cardiovascular assessments and sometimes interventions to prevent severe outcomes.

7. Autonomic Dysfunction:

Dysfunction of the autonomic nervous system, known as dysautonomia, is another common issue in EDS. Symptoms can include postural orthostatic tachycardia syndrome (POTS), which causes dizziness, fainting, and rapid heart rate upon standing, and can significantly impact daily activities.

8. Ocular Complications:

In some types of EDS, the eyes can be affected, leading to issues such as myopia (nearsightedness), retinal detachment, and blue sclera (a bluish tint to the whites of the eyes). These ocular symptoms necessitate regular ophthalmologic evaluations.

9. Dental and Oral Issues:

Individuals with EDS may have fragile gums and mucous membranes, leading to frequent oral ulcers and periodontal disease. Dental crowding and high palate are also common and can complicate oral health care.

10. Fatigue and General Well-being:

Chronic fatigue is a prevalent symptom in EDS, likely due to the constant strain on muscles and joints, pain, and sleep disturbances. Managing fatigue requires a comprehensive approach, including pacing activities, optimizing sleep, and addressing pain and other contributing factors.

The variability and complexity of EDS symptoms underscore the importance of a multidisciplinary approach to diagnosis and management. Each individual's experience with EDS is unique, requiring personalized care plans that address the specific manifestations and complications they face.

Ehlers-Danlos Syndrome (EDS) often coexists with a range of other conditions, known as comorbidities, which can complicate diagnosis and management. Understanding these co-existing conditions is essential for providing comprehensive care to individuals with EDS.

1. Mast Cell Activation Syndrome (MCAS):

MCAS is a condition characterized by inappropriate mast cell activation, leading to symptoms like flushing, hives, gastrointestinal distress, and anaphylaxis. People with EDS are at higher risk for MCAS, and the symptoms can overlap, making diagnosis challenging. Managing MCAS involves identifying and avoiding triggers, and using medications like antihistamines and mast cell stabilizers.

2. Dysautonomia and Postural Orthostatic Tachycardia Syndrome (POTS):

Dysautonomia, particularly POTS, is common in EDS patients. POTS causes a significant increase in heart rate upon standing, leading to dizziness, fatigue, and syncope (fainting). Management includes increasing fluid and salt intake, wearing compression garments, and using medications like beta-blockers or fludrocortisone to stabilize blood pressure and heart rate.

3. Chronic Pain and Fibromyalgia:

Chronic pain is a prevalent issue in EDS, often exacerbated by joint instability and repeated injuries. Fibromyalgia, a condition characterized by widespread musculoskeletal pain, is also common. Treatment involves a multidisciplinary approach, including physical therapy, pain medications, cognitive behavioral therapy, and alternative therapies such as acupuncture.

4. Gastrointestinal Disorders:

Gastrointestinal issues in EDS, such as IBS, GERD, and gastroparesis (delayed stomach emptying), require careful dietary management and sometimes medications to manage symptoms. Working with a gastroenterologist familiar with EDS can help tailor treatment plans effectively.

5. Mental Health Conditions:

Living with EDS and its associated challenges can lead to mental health issues such as anxiety, depression, and PTSD. Access to mental health professionals who understand the complexities of EDS is crucial. Cognitive behavioral therapy, support groups, and, when necessary, medications can help manage these conditions.

6. Sleep disorders:

Sleep disturbances, including insomnia and sleep apnea, are common in EDS. Addressing underlying causes such as pain and gastrointestinal issues, creating a conducive sleep environment, and using appropriate medications or devices like CPAP for sleep apnea can improve sleep quality.

7. Osteoporosis and Bone Health:

Individuals with EDS may be at increased risk for osteoporosis due to reduced bone density. Ensuring adequate calcium and vitamin D intake, weight-bearing exercises, and medications can help maintain bone health.

8. Temporomandibular Joint Disorders (TMJ):

TMJ disorders, causing jaw pain and dysfunction, are often seen in EDS due to joint laxity. Management includes physical therapy, dental interventions, and sometimes surgical options.

9. Pelvic and Bladder Issues:

Pelvic organ prolapses and bladder dysfunction, including interstitial cystitis, are common in EDS. Pelvic floor therapy and medications can help manage these symptoms.

10. Cardiovascular Issues:

Apart from vascular EDS, other cardiovascular issues like mitral valve prolapse and aortic root dilation require regular monitoring and sometimes surgical intervention to prevent complications.

Understanding the full spectrum of comorbidities and co-existing conditions in EDS is crucial for developing a holistic treatment plan. This comprehensive approach ensures that all aspects of a patient's health are addressed, improving their overall quality of life.

Collaboration among various specialists, patient education, and active self-management are key components of effectively managing EDS and its associated conditions.

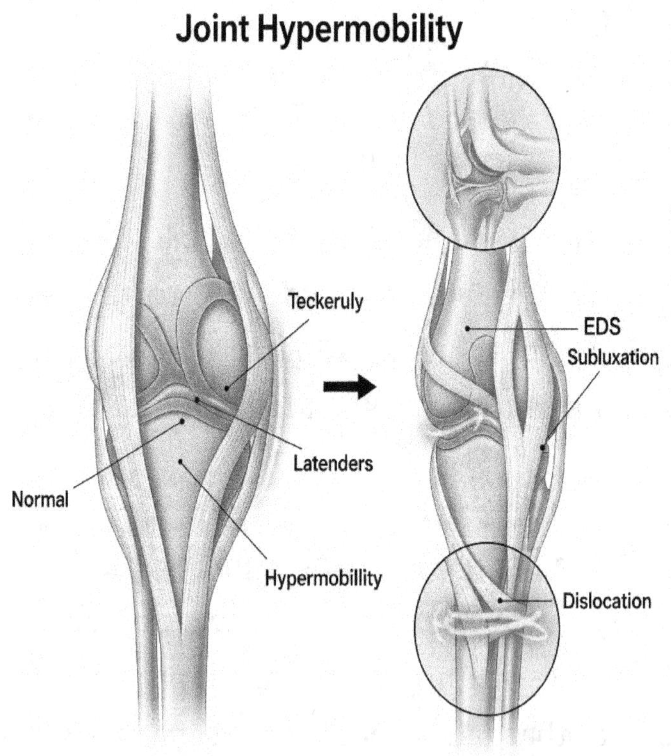

CHAPTER THREE

YOU ARE NOT ALONE: THE EDS COMMUNITY AND SUPPORT

3.1 Finding friends: Connecting with others who understand

Living with Ehlers-Danlos Syndrome (EDS) can sometimes feel isolating, especially when the condition is rare and misunderstood. However, finding a supportive community of individuals who share similar experiences can be incredibly empowering and validating. Here's why connecting with others who understand is essential for individuals with EDS:

1. Validation and Understanding:

Meeting others who are also living with EDS can provide a sense of validation and understanding that is difficult to find elsewhere. Sharing experiences, symptoms, and coping strategies with fellow EDS warriors can help individuals feel less alone and more understood.

2. Sharing Knowledge and Resources:

In a community of individuals with EDS, there is a wealth of knowledge and resources available. From practical tips for managing symptoms to recommendations for healthcare providers, support groups offer valuable insights that can significantly improve quality of life.

3. Emotional Support:

Living with a chronic condition like EDS can take a toll on mental and emotional wellbeing. Having a supportive community to lean on during difficult times can provide much-needed emotional support and encouragement. Knowing that others are facing similar challenges can foster a sense of solidarity and resilience.

4. Advocacy and Empowerment:

Collective advocacy is a powerful tool for raising awareness about EDS and advocating for better healthcare and support services. By connecting with others who understand the challenges of living with EDS, individuals can amplify their voices and work together to effect positive change in their communities and beyond.

5. Building Lifelong Friendships:

The bonds formed within the EDS community often extend beyond shared medical experiences. Many individuals forge lifelong friendships with others they meet through support groups and advocacy efforts. These friendships provide not only camaraderie but also practical support and companionship on the journey with EDS.

Finding your tribe within the EDS community can be a transformative experience, offering validation, support, and empowerment in the face of the challenges posed by the condition. Whether through local support groups, online communities, or advocacy organizations, connecting with others who understand can make a world of difference in navigating life with EDS.

In today's digital age, the internet has revolutionized the way individuals with chronic conditions like Ehlers-Danlos Syndrome (EDS) connect and support each other. Online support groups and forums offer a virtual space where individuals can share experiences, ask questions, and find encouragement from others who understand. Here's why online support groups are invaluable for individuals with EDS:

1. Accessibility and Convenience:

Online support groups and forums are accessible to individuals regardless of their location or mobility limitations. This accessibility makes it easier for individuals with EDS, who may struggle with mobility or transportation challenges, to connect with others and access support.

2. Anonymity and Privacy:

For some individuals with EDS, discussing personal experiences and symptoms openly can be intimidating. Online support groups provide a level of anonymity and privacy that allows individuals to share their stories and seek advice without fear of judgment or stigma.

3. Diverse Perspectives and Experiences:

Online support groups bring together individuals from diverse backgrounds and experiences, offering a broad range of perspectives and insights. This diversity enriches discussions and ensures that individuals can find support and advice that resonates with their unique circumstances.

4. 24/7 Support:

Living with a chronic condition like EDS means that symptoms and challenges can arise at any time. Online support groups provide a 24/7 support network, allowing individuals to seek advice, share concerns, or simply connect with others, no matter the time of day or night.

5. Expert Advice and Resources:

Many online support groups are moderated by healthcare professionals or individuals with expertise in EDS. These moderators can provide valuable guidance, answer medical questions, and share resources to help individuals better manage their condition.

6. Empowerment and Advocacy:

Online support groups often serve as platforms for advocacy and awareness-raising efforts. By sharing their stories and experiences online, individuals with EDS can raise awareness about the condition, advocate for better healthcare, and connect with policymakers and researchers.

7. Building Lasting Connections:

Online support groups have the potential to foster meaningful connections and friendships that extend beyond the digital realm. Many individuals form close bonds with others they meet online, providing ongoing support and companionship on their journey with EDS.

While online support groups cannot replace face-to-face interactions entirely, they offer a valuable complement to traditional support networks. For individuals with EDS, online communities provide a lifeline of support, information, and connection that can profoundly impact their wellbeing and quality of life. Whether seeking advice, sharing experiences, or offering encouragement, the power of online support groups lies in their ability to bring together individuals who understand and support each other on the journey with EDS.

3.3 Advocating for Yourself and the EDS Community

Advocacy plays a crucial role in raising awareness about Ehlers-Danlos Syndrome (EDS), improving access to quality healthcare, and fostering a supportive environment for individuals living with the condition. Here's why advocating for yourself and the EDS community is essential:

1. Raising Awareness:

Many people, including healthcare professionals, are unfamiliar with EDS or misunderstand its complexities. By sharing your story and raising awareness about EDS, you can help educate others and dispel misconceptions surrounding the condition.

2. Improving Access to Care:

Accessing appropriate healthcare and support services can be challenging for individuals with EDS. By advocating for better access to specialist care, diagnostic tools, and treatment options, you can help ensure that individuals with EDS receive the support and resources they need to manage their condition effectively.

3. Empowering Others:

Advocating for yourself and the EDS community empowers others to do the same. By speaking up about your experiences, challenges, and needs, you inspire others to advocate for themselves and seek the care and support they deserve.

4. Effecting Change:

Collective advocacy has the power to effect systemic change and improve outcomes for individuals with EDS. By joining forces with other advocates, participating in awareness campaigns, and engaging with policymakers and healthcare organizations, you can contribute to meaningful changes in the way EDS is understood and treated.

5. Creating Supportive Communities:

Advocacy efforts often lead to the creation of supportive communities and networks for individuals with EDS. By coming together to advocate for common goals, individuals can build strong, supportive communities that provide encouragement, resources, and solidarity.

6. Fostering Research and Innovation:

Advocacy plays a crucial role in driving research and innovation in the field of EDS. By advocating for increased funding for EDS research, participating in clinical trials, and sharing insights with researchers, individuals with EDS can contribute to advancements in understanding and treating the condition.

7. Amplifying Voices:

Every voice matters in the fight for better recognition and support for EDS. By amplifying your voice through advocacy efforts, you help ensure that the needs and experiences of individuals with EDS are heard and addressed by policymakers, healthcare providers, and society at large.

Advocating for yourself and the EDS community is a powerful way to make a difference in the lives of individuals living with the condition. Whether through raising awareness, improving access to care, or effecting systemic change, advocacy efforts have the potential to positively impact the wellbeing and quality of life of individuals with EDS and their families. By speaking up, sharing your story, and advocating for change, you can help build a brighter future for the EDS community.

CHAPTER FOUR

THE BODY IN MOTION: TAILORED EXERCISE FOR EDS

4.1 Why Movement Matters: The Importance of Exercise for Overall Wellbeing

Movement is fundamental to human health, and for individuals with Ehlers-Danlos Syndrome (EDS), exercise plays a particularly vital role in maintaining and enhancing overall wellbeing. The benefits of physical activity extend beyond mere fitness; they encompass improved joint stability, enhanced muscle strength, and better mental health.

Strengthening Muscles and Stabilizing Joints:

One of the primary reasons exercises is crucial for people with EDS is its role in strengthening muscles that support and stabilize hypermobile joints. Stronger muscles can compensate for the laxity of connective tissues, reducing the likelihood of dislocations and subluxations. This stabilization can lead to a significant reduction in pain and an improvement in functional abilities.

Improving Cardiovascular Health:

Regular physical activity enhances cardiovascular health, which is particularly important for individuals with EDS who might be prone to conditions like POTS (Postural Orthostatic Tachycardia Syndrome). Cardiovascular exercises, such as walking, swimming, or cycling, help improve heart rate variability and blood circulation, reducing symptoms of dizziness and fatigue associated with autonomic dysfunction.

Enhancing Mental Health:

The benefits of exercise on mental health are well-documented. For those living with EDS, regular physical activity can alleviate symptoms of anxiety and depression, enhance mood, and improve overall quality of life. Exercise triggers the release of endorphins, the body's natural painkillers, and mood elevators, which can be particularly beneficial for managing chronic pain and emotional stress.

Maintaining Flexibility and Mobility:

While hypermobility is a characteristic feature of EDS, maintaining a healthy range of motion is still important. Controlled, gentle stretching exercises can help maintain flexibility without overstressing joints. This balance is crucial to avoid exacerbating joint instability while ensuring that muscles remain supple and functional.

Preventing Deconditioning:

A sedentary lifestyle can lead to deconditioning, where muscles weaken, and cardiovascular fitness declines. This can create a vicious cycle of decreased activity leading to increased pain and disability. Regular exercise helps break this cycle, promoting a more active lifestyle that supports overall health and wellbeing.

Promoting Bone Health:

Weight-bearing exercises, even at a low impact, are essential for maintaining bone density. This is particularly important for individuals with EDS, who may be at an increased risk of osteoporosis due to chronic joint instability and reduced physical activity.

Personal Empowerment and Control:

Exercise provides a sense of control and empowerment, allowing individuals with EDS to actively participate in their health management. Setting achievable fitness goals and seeing progress can boost self-esteem and provide motivation to continue engaging in physical activity.

Understanding the unique needs and limitations of the body is critical when designing an exercise regimen for EDS. It is essential to work with healthcare professionals, such as physical therapists and fitness trainers experienced with EDS, to develop a personalized and safe exercise plan that addresses individual capabilities and goals.

4.2 Finding Your Perfect Fit: Exploring Low-Impact and Gentle Exercise Options

For individuals with EDS, high-impact activities and intense workouts may not be suitable due to the risk of joint damage and injury. Instead, low-impact and gentle exercise options provide safe and effective ways to stay active and healthy. Finding the perfect fit involves exploring various activities that cater to the unique needs of EDS patients.

Swimming and Aquatic Therapy:

Water-based exercises are highly recommended for individuals with EDS. The buoyancy of water reduces stress on joints while providing resistance that helps strengthen muscles. Swimming, water aerobics, and aquatic therapy sessions can improve cardiovascular health, muscle tone, and flexibility without risking joint injury. The water's resistance also helps enhance muscle endurance and overall fitness.

Yoga and Pilates:

Yoga and Pilates focus on controlled movements, flexibility, and core strength, making them ideal for people with EDS. These practices emphasize proper alignment and breathing techniques, which can help stabilize joints and improve posture. Modifications can be made to traditional poses to accommodate individual limitations, ensuring a safe and beneficial practice. Additionally, the mindfulness aspect of yoga can aid in managing stress and improving mental health.

Tai Chi and Qigong:

Tai Chi and Qigong are ancient Chinese practices that involve slow, deliberate movements and deep breathing. These low-impact exercises enhance balance, flexibility, and muscle strength. The meditative aspect of these practices also promotes relaxation and stress reduction, which can be particularly beneficial for managing the mental and emotional aspects of living with EDS.

Cycling:

Stationary or recumbent cycling provides an excellent cardiovascular workout with minimal impact on the joints. Cycling helps strengthen the lower body muscles and improve cardiovascular fitness. For those with EDS, using a stationary bike reduces the risk of falls and allows for controlled resistance levels, making it a safe and effective exercise option.

Strength Training with Resistance Bands:

Strength training is essential for building muscle support around hypermobile joints. Using resistance bands allows for controlled, low-impact strength training that can be easily adjusted to individual fitness levels. Focusing on slow, deliberate movements ensures that muscles are engaged without putting undue stress on the joints.

Walking:

Walking is a simple yet effective low-impact exercise that can be easily incorporated into daily routines. It improves cardiovascular health, muscle strength, and joint mobility. Using supportive footwear and walking on even surfaces can minimize the risk of injury. Gradually increasing walking duration and intensity can help build endurance and overall fitness.

Stretching and Flexibility Exercises:

Gentle stretching exercises help maintain flexibility and prevent muscle tightness. It's essential to avoid overstretching hypermobile joints, so stretches should be performed with caution and within a comfortable range of motion. Incorporating regular stretching routines can enhance mobility and reduce muscle stiffness.

Chair Exercises:

For individuals with significant mobility limitations, chair exercises provide a safe and effective way to stay active. These exercises can include seated strength training, stretching, and cardiovascular activities. Chair exercises can be adapted to various fitness levels and help maintain muscle tone and flexibility without placing stress on the joints.

Dance Therapy:

Dance therapy combines movement with music and can be adapted to suit different levels of mobility. It provides a fun and engaging way to improve cardiovascular fitness, coordination, and muscle strength. Dance movements can be modified to ensure safety and comfort, making it a versatile exercise option for people with EDS.

Exploring these low-impact and gentle exercise options allows individuals with EDS to find activities they enjoy and can sustain long-term. Working with a physical therapist or exercise specialist familiar with EDS can help tailor an exercise program that meets individual needs and goals, ensuring safety and effectiveness.

Creating a sustainable exercise routine is essential for individuals with EDS to maintain their health and wellbeing. A well-designed routine should be tailored to individual capabilities, preferences, and goals, ensuring that exercise becomes a regular and enjoyable part of life.

Setting Realistic Goals:

Establishing achievable and realistic fitness goals is the first step in creating a sustainable exercise routine. Goals should be specific, measurable, and tailored to individual needs. For example, improving joint stability, increasing muscle strength, or enhancing cardiovascular fitness. Breaking down long-term goals into smaller, manageable milestones can provide a sense of accomplishment and motivation.

Incorporating Variety:

Variety is key to preventing boredom and maintaining motivation. Incorporating different types of exercises, such as swimming, yoga, cycling, and strength training, can keep the routine interesting and engaging. Mixing up activities also ensures a comprehensive workout that addresses various aspects of fitness, including strength, flexibility, and cardiovascular health.

Scheduling Regular Exercise:

Consistency is crucial for reaping the benefits of exercise. Scheduling regular workout sessions and treating them as non-negotiable appointments can help establish a routine. Finding the best time of day to exercise, whether it's morning, afternoon, or evening, can make it easier to stick to the routine. It's also important to listen to the body and allow for flexibility on days when symptoms may flare up.

Pacing and Rest:

Pacing is vital for individuals with EDS to avoid overexertion and injury. Gradually increasing the intensity and duration of exercise allows the body to adapt without causing stress to the joints and muscles. Incorporating rest days and recovery periods into the routine ensures that the body has time to heal and rebuild. Understanding the balance between activity and rest can prevent setbacks and promote long-term adherence to the exercise plan.

Using Proper Equipment and Support:

Using appropriate equipment and support can enhance the safety and effectiveness of exercise routines. Supportive footwear, braces, and orthotics can provide additional stability during physical activities. Resistance bands, lightweight dumbbells, and other exercise tools can be used to perform strength training exercises safely. Consulting with a physical therapist can help identify the best equipment for individual needs.

Tracking Progress:

Keeping a record of exercise activities, including the type, duration, and intensity, can help track progress and identify patterns. Monitoring improvements in strength, flexibility, and overall fitness provides motivation and a sense of achievement. Tracking can also help identify any adjustments needed in the routine to ensure it remains effective and enjoyable.

Staying Motivated:

Maintaining motivation is crucial for long-term adherence to an exercise routine. Finding activities that are enjoyable and fulfilling can make exercise feel less like a chore and more like a rewarding experience. Setting new challenges, such as participating in a charity walk or learning a new yoga pose, can keep the routine exciting. Joining a support group or exercising with a friend can provide additional motivation and accountability.

Adapting to Changes:

Flexibility and adaptability are essential for sustaining an exercise routine. Symptoms of EDS can vary, and it's important to adjust the routine based on how the body feels. On days when symptoms are more severe, opting for gentler activities or focusing on stretching and relaxation can ensure continued movement without causing harm. Recognizing and respecting the body's limits is key to maintaining a healthy and sustainable exercise regimen.

Creating a sustainable exercise routine involves careful planning, setting realistic goals, and incorporating variety and flexibility. By moving with intention and understanding the unique needs of the body, individuals with EDS can enjoy the numerous benefits of regular physical activity while minimizing the risk of injury and promoting long-term health and wellbeing.

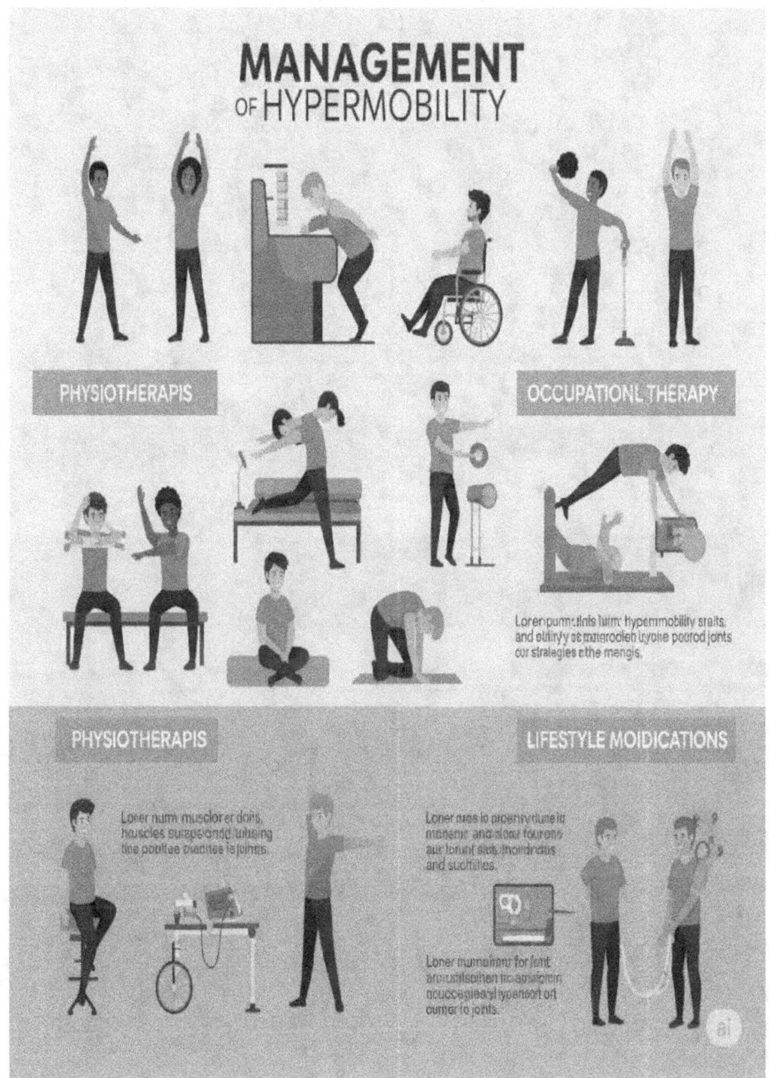

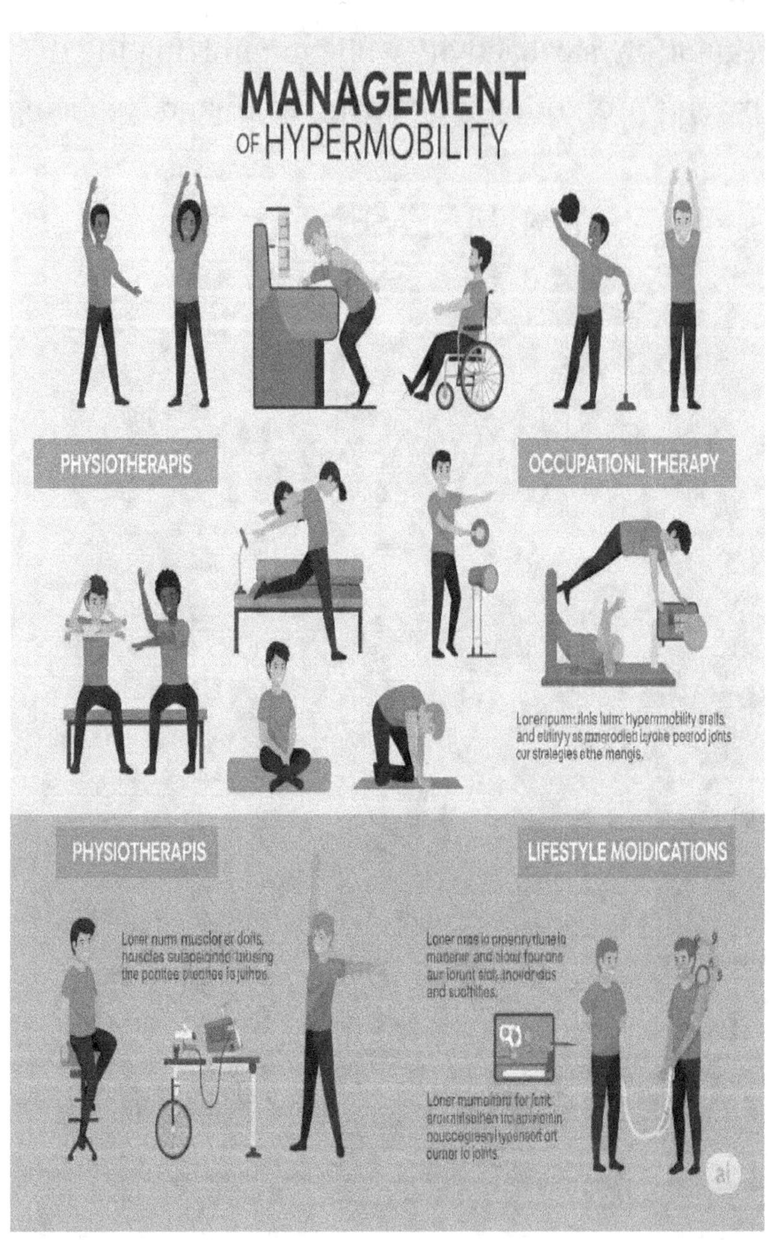

MANAGEMENT
OF HYPERMOBILITY
PHYSIOTHERAPIS
OCCUPATIONL THERAPY
PHYSIOTHERAPIS
LIFESTYLE MOIDICATIONS

CHAPTER FIVE

FUELING YOUR BODY FOR SUCCESS: NUTRITION FOR EDS

5.1 Understanding Your Nutritional Needs: Dietary Considerations for EDS

Nutrition plays a pivotal role in managing Ehlers-Danlos Syndrome (EDS) and optimizing overall health and wellbeing. Understanding your nutritional needs and making informed dietary choices can help alleviate symptoms, support healing, and enhance your quality of life with EDS. Here's what you need to know about dietary considerations for EDS:

1. Nutrient-Rich Foods:

A diet rich in nutrients is essential for individuals with EDS to support optimal health and manage symptoms effectively. Focus on incorporating a variety of nutrient-dense foods into your diet, including fruits, vegetables, whole grains, lean proteins, and healthy fats.

2. Anti-Inflammatory Foods:

Inflammation is a common feature of EDS and can exacerbate symptoms such as joint pain and fatigue. Incorporating anti-inflammatory foods into your diet, such as fatty fish, leafy greens, berries, nuts, and seeds, can help reduce inflammation and alleviate symptoms.

3. Hydration:

Proper hydration is crucial for individuals with EDS, as dehydration can exacerbate symptoms such as headaches, fatigue, and muscle cramps. Aim to drink plenty of water throughout the day and consider incorporating hydrating foods such as fruits and vegetables into your diet.

4. Adequate Protein Intake:

Protein is essential for supporting muscle strength and repair, which is particularly important for individuals with EDS who may experience muscle weakness and joint instability. Ensure that you consume an adequate amount of protein from sources such as lean meats, poultry, fish, eggs, dairy products, legumes, and plant-based alternatives.

5. Calcium and Vitamin D:

Bone and joint health are of particular concern for individuals with EDS due to the risk of osteoporosis and joint dislocations. Ensure that your diet includes sufficient calcium and vitamin D, which are essential for bone strength and density. Good dietary sources of calcium include dairy products, leafy greens, fortified foods, and supplements if necessary.

6. Individualized Approach:

Every individual with EDS is unique, and dietary needs can vary based on factors such as age, gender, activity level, and specific symptoms. Work with a healthcare professional, such as a registered dietitian or nutritionist, to develop a personalized nutrition plan that meets your individual needs and addresses any dietary restrictions or challenges you may face.

Understanding your nutritional needs and making informed dietary choices can empower you to take control of your health and manage your EDS more effectively. By nourishing your body with nutrient-rich foods, prioritizing hydration, and addressing any specific dietary considerations, you can support your overall wellbeing and thrive despite the challenges of living with EDS.

5.2 Building a Balanced Plate: Optimizing Your Diet for Energy and Wellbeing

Maintaining a balanced and nutritious diet is essential for individuals with Ehlers-Danlos Syndrome (EDS) to support optimal energy levels, manage symptoms effectively, and promote overall wellbeing. Building a balanced plate involves selecting a variety of nutrient-dense foods from different food groups to ensure that your body receives the essential nutrients it needs. Here are some tips for optimizing your diet for energy and wellbeing with EDS:

1. Include a Variety of Foods:

Aim to include a diverse range of foods from all food groups in your meals and snacks. Incorporate plenty of fruits, vegetables, whole grains, lean proteins, and healthy fats to provide your body with a wide array of essential nutrients.

2. Prioritize Whole Foods:

Choose whole, minimally processed foods whenever possible, as they tend to be higher in nutrients and lower in added sugars, unhealthy fats, and artificial additives. Fill your plate with whole grains, fresh fruits and vegetables, lean proteins, and healthy fats to support optimal health and energy levels.

3. Pay Attention to Portions:

Maintaining appropriate portion sizes is important for managing weight and energy levels, especially for individuals with EDS who may have fluctuations in appetite and metabolism. Use portion control strategies such as measuring serving sizes, eating mindfully, and paying attention to hunger and fullness cues.

4. Balance Macronutrients:

Ensure that your meals and snacks contain a balance of carbohydrates, proteins, and fats to provide sustained energy and support overall health. Aim to include complex carbohydrates, lean proteins, and healthy fats in each meal to help stabilize blood sugar levels and promote satiety.

5. Stay Hydrated:

Proper hydration is crucial for maintaining energy levels, supporting digestion, and promoting overall health. Drink plenty of water throughout the day and consider incorporating hydrating beverages such as herbal tea, coconut water, and infused water into your routine.

6. Listen to Your Body:

Pay attention to how different foods make you feel and adjust your diet accordingly. Keep a food diary to track your intake and any associated symptoms or reactions, and use this information to identify foods that support your energy and wellbeing and those that may exacerbate symptoms.

By building a balanced plate with a variety of nutrient-rich foods, prioritizing whole foods, paying attention to portions, balancing macronutrients, staying hydrated, and listening to your body, you can optimize your diet to support energy levels, manage symptoms, and promote overall wellbeing with EDS.

5.3 Addressing Digestive Challenges: Strategies for Managing Gut Issues in EDS

Digestive challenges are common among individuals with Ehlers-Danlos Syndrome (EDS) and can significantly impact quality of life. From gastrointestinal symptoms such as reflux and constipation to more complex conditions like irritable bowel syndrome (IBS) and gastroparesis, managing gut issues is an important aspect of EDS management. Here are some strategies for addressing digestive challenges and managing gut issues in EDS:

1. Maintain a Digestive Diary:

Keeping track of your symptoms, diet, and lifestyle factors in a digestive diary can help you identify patterns and triggers related to your gut issues. Record what you eat, when you eat it, and any symptoms or reactions you experience to pinpoint potential food sensitivities or exacerbating factors.

2. Follow a Gut-Friendly Diet:

Adopting a gut-friendly diet can help alleviate digestive symptoms and support gut health. Focus on incorporating fiber-rich foods, such as fruits, vegetables, whole grains, and legumes, to promote regularity and bowel function. Limiting trigger foods such as spicy foods, caffeine, alcohol, and processed foods may also help reduce digestive discomfort.

3. Support Digestive Function:

Supporting digestive function with lifestyle modifications and natural remedies can help manage gut issues in EDS. Practice mindful eating, chew food thoroughly, and eat smaller, more frequent meals to ease digestion. Incorporate gut-supportive supplements such as probiotics, digestive enzymes, and fiber supplements under the guidance of a healthcare professional.

4. Manage Stress:

Stress can exacerbate digestive symptoms and contribute to gut issues in EDS. Incorporate stress-management techniques such as deep breathing, meditation, yoga, and progressive muscle relaxation into your daily routine to promote relaxation and reduce stress-related gut symptoms.

5. Stay Hydrated:

Proper hydration is essential for maintaining digestive health and supporting regular bowel function. Drink plenty of water throughout the day to prevent dehydration and promote optimal digestion and nutrient absorption.

6. Seek Medical Guidance:

If you experience persistent or severe digestive symptoms, consult with a healthcare professional for a comprehensive evaluation and personalized treatment plan. Your healthcare provider can help identify underlying digestive conditions, prescribe appropriate medications, and recommend dietary and lifestyle modifications to manage your gut issues effectively.

By maintaining a digestive diary, following a gut-friendly diet, supporting digestive function, managing stress, staying hydrated, and seeking medical guidance when needed, you can address digestive challenges and manage gut issues effectively as part of your EDS management plan.

CHAPTER SIX

SLEEP, THE BODY'S RESTORATIVE POWERHOUSE

6.1 The Importance of Quality Sleep in Managing EDS Symptoms

Quality sleep is a cornerstone of managing Ehlers-Danlos Syndrome (EDS) symptoms effectively. Sleep is when the body repairs, restores, and rejuvenates itself, playing a vital role in overall health and wellbeing. For individuals with EDS, prioritizing quality sleep is particularly important due to the impact of the condition on physical and mental health. Here's why quality sleep matters in managing EDS symptoms:

1. Tissue Repair and Healing:

During sleep, the body undergoes essential processes of tissue repair and healing. Adequate sleep allows for the repair of damaged connective tissues, muscles, and ligaments, which can help alleviate symptoms such as joint pain and instability associated with EDS.

2. Pain Management:

Quality sleep plays a crucial role in pain management for individuals with EDS. Poor sleep can exacerbate pain sensitivity and perception, leading to increased discomfort and reduced quality of life. By prioritizing quality sleep, individuals with EDS can better manage pain symptoms and improve their overall wellbeing.

3. Energy Restoration:

EDS often causes fatigue and low energy levels due to factors such as poor sleep quality, disrupted sleep patterns, and underlying medical conditions. Quality sleep allows for the restoration of energy levels, helping individuals with EDS feel more refreshed, alert, and capable of managing daily activities.

4. Immune Function:

Sleep is essential for maintaining a healthy immune system, which is particularly important for individuals with EDS who may be more susceptible to infections and illnesses. Adequate sleep supports immune function, helping to prevent infections and promote overall health and wellbeing.

5. Mental Health:

Quality sleep is closely linked to mental health and emotional wellbeing. Poor sleep can contribute to mood disturbances, anxiety, and depression, which are common challenges faced by individuals with EDS. Prioritizing quality sleep can help improve mood, reduce stress, and enhance overall mental health.

6. Cognitive Function:

Sleep plays a crucial role in cognitive function, including memory consolidation, learning, and decision-making. Individuals with EDS may experience cognitive difficulties such as brain fog and concentration problems, which can be exacerbated by poor sleep. Quality sleep supports optimal cognitive function, helping individuals with EDS think more clearly and function more effectively.

By recognizing the importance of quality sleep in managing EDS symptoms, individuals can take proactive steps to prioritize sleep hygiene, address sleep disturbances, and optimize their sleep environment for restorative rest.

Creating a sleep sanctuary is essential for individuals with Ehlers-Danlos Syndrome (EDS) to optimize their sleep environment and promote restful nights. A sleep sanctuary is a calm, comfortable, and supportive space designed to facilitate quality sleep and minimize sleep disturbances. Here are some tips for creating a sleep sanctuary and optimizing your sleep environment:

1. Comfortable Mattress and Bedding:

Invest in a comfortable mattress and high-quality bedding that provides adequate support and promotes proper alignment of the spine and joints. Choose a mattress and pillows that suit your individual comfort preferences and provide relief for pressure points and areas of pain or discomfort.

2. Temperature Control:

Maintain a comfortable temperature in your sleep environment, keeping it cool and well-ventilated to promote restful sleep. Use bedding materials and sleepwear that allow for temperature regulation, and consider using a fan, air conditioner, or humidifier to create optimal sleeping conditions.

3. Light Management:

Create a dark and conducive sleep environment by minimizing exposure to light sources such as electronic devices, streetlights, and ambient light from outside. Use blackout curtains or shades to block out unwanted light and consider using a sleep mask if necessary to further enhance darkness.

4. Noise Reduction:

Minimize noise disturbances in your sleep environment by using earplugs, white noise machines, or soundproofing materials to block out unwanted sounds. Create a quiet and peaceful atmosphere conducive to restful sleep, and consider using relaxation techniques such as deep breathing or meditation to promote relaxation and reduce stress.

5. Declutter and Personalize:

Create a clutter-free and personalized sleep environment that promotes feelings of calmness and relaxation. Remove clutter and unnecessary items from your bedroom, and decorate with soothing colors, textures, and decor that evoke feelings of tranquility and serenity.

6. Establish a Bedtime Routine:

Establish a consistent bedtime routine to signal to your body that it's time to wind down and prepare for sleep. Engage in relaxing activities such as reading, listening to calming music, or taking a warm bath to help promote relaxation and cue your body for sleep.

By creating a sleep sanctuary and optimizing your sleep environment for restful nights, you can enhance the quality of your sleep and improve your overall wellbeing with EDS.

6.3 Developing Healthy Sleep Habits: Strategies for Falling Asleep and Staying Asleep

Developing healthy sleep habits is essential for individuals with Ehlers-Danlos Syndrome (EDS) to improve the quality and duration of their sleep and manage symptoms effectively. Healthy sleep habits, also known as sleep hygiene, involve adopting practices and behaviors that promote restful sleep and support optimal sleep quality. Here are some strategies for developing healthy sleep habits and improving sleep with EDS:

1. Maintain a Consistent Sleep Schedule:

Establish a regular sleep-wake schedule by going to bed and waking up at the same time every day, even on weekends. Consistency helps regulate your body's internal clock and promotes better sleep quality and duration.

2. Create a Relaxing Bedtime Routine:

Develop a relaxing bedtime routine to unwind and prepare your body and mind for sleep. Engage in calming activities such as reading, practicing gentle yoga or stretching, or taking a warm bath to promote relaxation and signal to your body that it's time to sleep.

3. Limit Exposure to Screens Before Bed:

Reduce exposure to electronic devices such as smartphones, tablets, computers, and televisions before bedtime, as the blue light emitted from screens can interfere with your body's natural sleep-wake cycle and make it harder to fall asleep. Aim to power down electronics at least an hour before bedtime to promote better sleep.

4. Create a Comfortable Sleep Environment:

Optimize your sleep environment to make it conducive to restful sleep. Ensure your bedroom is dark, quiet, and comfortably cool, and invest in a comfortable mattress, supportive pillows, and high-quality bedding to enhance sleep comfort and quality.

5. Limit Stimulants and Heavy Meals Before Bed:

Avoid consuming stimulants such as caffeine and nicotine in the hours leading up to bedtime, as they can interfere with your ability to fall asleep. Additionally, avoid heavy meals and large amounts of liquids close to bedtime to prevent discomfort and disruptions to sleep.

6. Manage Stress and Anxiety:

Practice stress-reduction techniques such as deep breathing, meditation, progressive muscle relaxation, or visualization exercises to calm your mind and body before bedtime. Managing stress and anxiety can help promote relaxation and improve sleep quality with EDS.

7. Get Regular Exercise:

Engage in regular physical activity or exercise during the day to promote better sleep at night. Aim for at least 30 minutes of moderate exercise most days of the week, but avoid vigorous exercise close to bedtime, as it can be stimulating and make it harder to fall asleep.

8. Seek Professional Help if Needed:

If you continue to experience difficulties falling asleep or staying asleep despite implementing healthy sleep habits, consider seeking guidance from a healthcare professional or sleep specialist. They can help identify underlying sleep disorders or issues contributing to sleep disturbances and recommend appropriate interventions or treatments.

By incorporating these healthy sleep habits into your daily routine, you can improve the quality and duration of your sleep, manage symptoms more effectively, and enhance your overall health and wellbeing with EDS.

CHAPTER SEVEN

TAMING THE PAIN: EFFECTIVE PAIN MANAGEMENT STRATEGIES

7.1 Understanding Different Types of Pain in EDS

Pain is a complex and multifaceted aspect of Ehlers-Danlos Syndrome (EDS), varying in type, severity, and frequency among individuals. Understanding the different types of pain associated with EDS is crucial for effective pain management. Here are some common types of pain experienced by individuals with EDS:

1. Joint Pain:

Joint pain is one of the hallmark symptoms of EDS and often affects the hypermobile joints characteristic of the condition. Individuals may experience pain, stiffness, swelling, and instability in affected joints, which can impact mobility and daily activities.

2. Musculoskeletal Pain:

Musculoskeletal pain refers to discomfort or tenderness in muscles, ligaments, and tendons, which are commonly affected in EDS due to the laxity and fragility of connective tissues. Musculoskeletal pain may present as muscle spasms, cramps, or generalized soreness.

3. Chronic Pain:

Chronic pain is persistent pain that lasts for an extended period, typically three months or longer. Many individuals with EDS experience chronic pain due to ongoing joint instability, tissue fragility, and other associated conditions such as fibromyalgia or neuropathic pain syndromes.

4. Neuropathic Pain:

Neuropathic pain results from damage or dysfunction of the nervous system and can manifest as shooting, burning, or tingling sensations. Neuropathic pain is common in individuals with EDS due to nerve compression, entrapment, or irritation caused by lax connective tissues or structural abnormalities.

5. Headaches and Migraines:

Headaches and migraines are prevalent in individuals with EDS and can be triggered by factors such as cervical instability, cranial settling, temporomandibular joint dysfunction (TMJ), or dysautonomia. These headaches may be debilitating and significantly impact quality of life.

6. Visceral Pain:

Visceral pain originates from internal organs and may present as abdominal pain, pelvic pain, or chest pain. Visceral pain in EDS can be associated with gastrointestinal issues such as gastroesophageal reflux disease (GERD), irritable bowel syndrome (IBS), or pelvic floor dysfunction.

Understanding the different types of pain experienced in EDS is essential for tailoring effective pain management strategies to address individual needs and symptoms. By identifying the specific characteristics and triggers of pain, individuals can work with healthcare providers to develop personalized treatment plans that aim to alleviate discomfort, improve function, and enhance quality of life.

7.2 Exploring Pain Management Options: Medication, Physical Therapy, and Alternative Therapies

Managing pain effectively in Ehlers-Danlos Syndrome (EDS) often requires a multimodal approach that combines various treatment modalities to address different aspects of pain and promote overall wellbeing. Here are some commonly used pains management options for individuals with EDS:

1. Medication:

Medications such as nonsteroidal anti-inflammatory drugs (NSAIDs), acetaminophen, or prescription pain relievers may be used to alleviate pain and reduce inflammation associated with EDS. However, long-term use of certain medications should be carefully monitored due to potential side effects and risks.

2. Physical Therapy:

Physical therapy plays a crucial role in managing pain and improving function in individuals with EDS. A physical therapist can design a personalized exercise program focused on strengthening muscles, stabilizing joints, improving flexibility, and promoting proper body mechanics to reduce pain and prevent injury.

3. Occupational Therapy:

Occupational therapy may be beneficial for individuals with EDS to learn adaptive strategies, ergonomic principles, and joint protection techniques to minimize pain and maximize independence in daily activities. Occupational therapists can provide assistive devices, splints, or modifications to support functional abilities.

4. Manual Therapy:

Manual therapy techniques such as massage therapy, chiropractic care, or osteopathic manipulation may offer temporary relief from musculoskeletal pain and tension in individuals with EDS. However, caution should be exercised to avoid excessive manipulation or hyperextension of fragile joints.

5. Alternative Therapies:

Complementary and alternative therapies such as acupuncture, acupressure, hydrotherapy, or transcutaneous electrical nerve stimulation (TENS) may provide additional pain relief and promote relaxation in individuals with EDS. These therapies can be used in conjunction with conventional treatments to address pain from multiple angles.

6. Psychological Interventions:

Psychological interventions such as cognitive-behavioral therapy (CBT), mindfulness-based stress reduction (MBSR), or relaxation techniques can help individuals with EDS cope with chronic pain, reduce stress, and improve emotional wellbeing. Addressing the psychological impact of pain is essential for holistic pain management.

7. Nutritional and Lifestyle Modifications:

Nutritional supplements, dietary modifications, and lifestyle changes such as stress management, adequate hydration, and regular physical activity can support overall health and reduce pain and inflammation in individuals with EDS. Consulting with a healthcare provider or registered dietitian is recommended for personalized guidance.

8. Pain Education and Self-Management:

Pain education programs and self-management strategies empower individuals with EDS to take an active role in managing their pain and improving quality of life. Learning about pain neuroscience, pacing techniques, relaxation strategies, and flare-up management can help individuals develop resilience and confidence in managing pain.

Exploring a combination of these pain management options tailored to individual needs and preferences can help individuals with EDS effectively manage pain, enhance function, and improve overall quality of life. Collaborating with a multidisciplinary healthcare team can provide comprehensive support and guidance in navigating the complexities of pain management in EDS.

7.3 Developing a Personalized Pain Management Plan

Developing a personalized pain management plan is essential for individuals with Ehlers-Danlos Syndrome (EDS) to address the unique challenges and symptoms associated with chronic pain effectively. A personalized pain management plan takes into account individual needs, preferences, and goals while incorporating a combination of treatment modalities to optimize pain relief and improve overall quality of life. Here are some key steps in developing a personalized pain management plan for EDS:

1. Comprehensive Assessment:

Start by conducting a comprehensive assessment of pain symptoms, triggers, severity, and impact on daily functioning. Work closely with healthcare providers, including primary care physicians, pain specialists, and allied health professionals, to gather information and identify underlying factors contributing to pain.

2. Set Realistic Goals:

Establish realistic and achievable goals for pain management based on individual needs and priorities. Goals may include reducing pain intensity, improving physical function and mobility, enhancing quality of life, and minimizing reliance on pain medications or invasive interventions.

3. Multimodal Approach:

Adopt a multimodal approach to pain management that integrates various treatment modalities to address different aspects of pain and promote overall wellbeing. Consider combining pharmacological interventions, physical therapy, psychological interventions, lifestyle modifications, and complementary therapies for comprehensive care.

4. Tailored Interventions:

Tailor interventions to individual needs and preferences while considering the specific challenges and comorbidities associated with EDS. Customize treatment plans to address hypermobility, joint instability, tissue fragility, autonomic dysfunction, and other underlying factors contributing to pain.

5. Collaborative Care:

Collaborate with a multidisciplinary healthcare team to coordinate care, monitor progress, and adjust treatment strategies as needed. Engage in shared decision-making and open communication with healthcare providers to ensure continuity of care and optimize outcomes.

6. Regular Monitoring and Evaluation:

Regularly monitor pain symptoms, treatment efficacy, and functional outcomes to evaluate progress and make necessary adjustments to the pain management plan. Track changes in pain intensity, activity levels, sleep quality, mood, and medication use to identify trends and patterns over time.

7. Patient Education and Empowerment:

Educate patients about pain neuroscience, self-management strategies, lifestyle modifications, and resources available for support. Empower patients to take an active role in managing their pain, making informed decisions, and advocating for their needs in healthcare settings.

8. Long-Term Follow-Up and Support:

Provide ongoing support, encouragement, and guidance to individuals with EDS as they navigate their pain management journey. Offer long-term follow-up care, access to support groups, and referrals to community resources to promote continuity of care and enhance resilience.

By following these steps and collaborating with healthcare providers, individuals with EDS can develop a personalized pain management plan that addresses their unique needs, improves symptom management, and enhances overall quality of life. Remember that pain management is an ongoing process that requires patience, persistence, and proactive self-care strategies.

Personalized Pain Management Plan
Ehlers-Danlos Syndrome

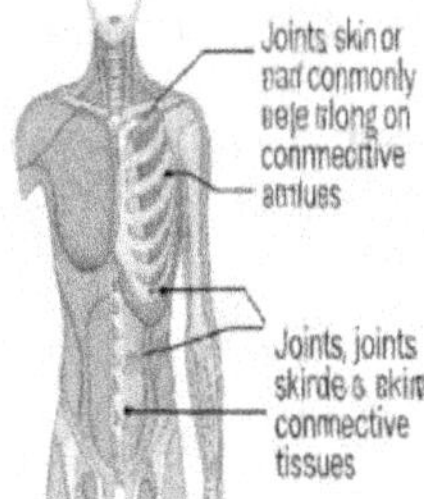

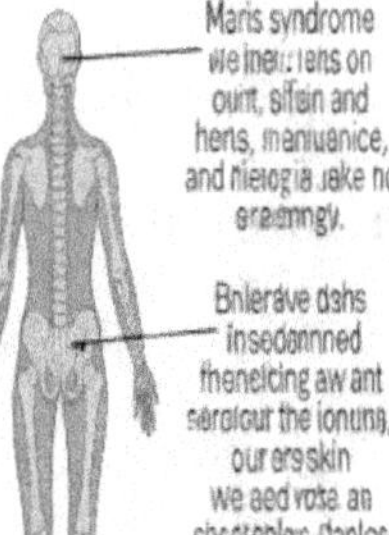

Physical Therapy

Mindfuless Techniques

Mindfuless Techniques

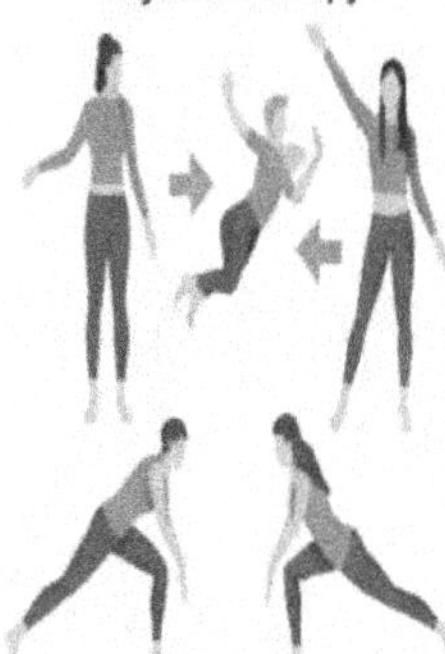

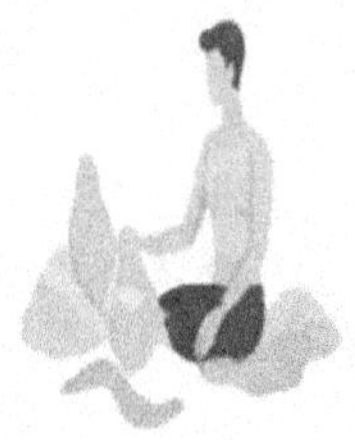

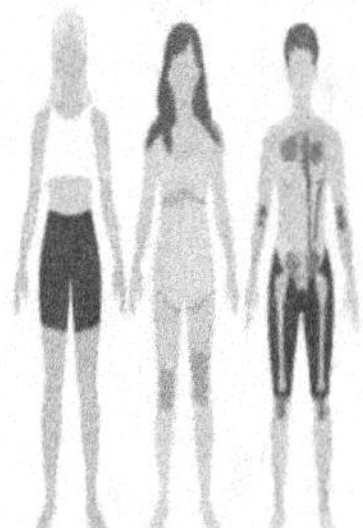

Modified Activities

Ergnomic Solutions

Dietary Advice

Medications

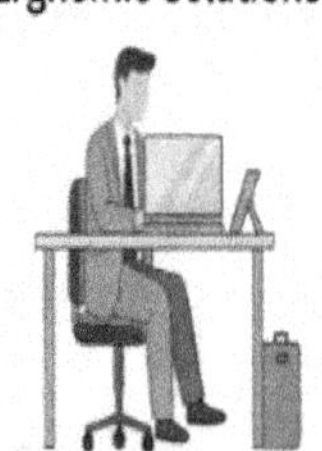

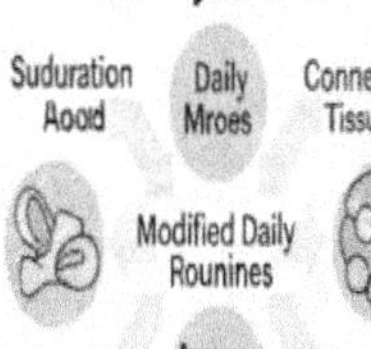

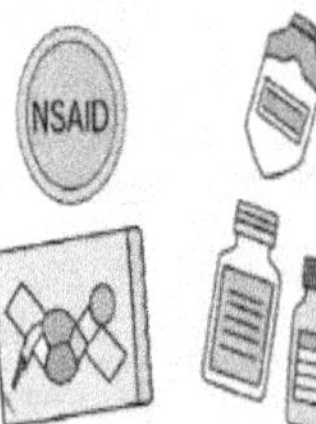

CHAPTER EIGHT

STRESS LESS, LIVE MORE: MANAGING STRESS AND EMOTIONAL WELLBEING

8.1 The Impact of Stress on EDS Symptoms: The Mind-Body Connection

Stress is an inevitable part of life, but for individuals with Ehlers-Danlos Syndrome (EDS), managing stress is particularly important due to its significant impact on symptoms and overall wellbeing. The mind-body connection plays a crucial role in how stress affects EDS symptoms. Here's how stress influences EDS:

1. Amplification of Symptoms:

Stress can exacerbate existing EDS symptoms, such as pain, fatigue, joint instability, and gastrointestinal issues. Heightened stress levels can intensify discomfort and impair daily functioning, making it challenging to manage the demands of everyday life.

2. Muscle Tension and Joint Strain:

Stress often leads to muscle tension and increased muscle guarding, which can contribute to joint strain and exacerbate hypermobility and instability in individuals with EDS. Chronic stress may worsen joint pain, stiffness, and mobility issues, further compromising physical function.

3. Dysregulation of the Nervous System:

Chronic stress can dysregulate the autonomic nervous system (ANS), leading to increased sympathetic activity ("fight or flight" response) and decreased parasympathetic activity ("rest and digest" response). This dysregulation may contribute to dysautonomia symptoms commonly experienced by individuals with EDS, such as dizziness, palpitations, and temperature intolerance.

4. Impaired Coping Mechanisms:

Living with a chronic and often unpredictable condition like EDS can be inherently stressful, leading to feelings of anxiety, frustration, and overwhelm. Stress may interfere with adaptive coping mechanisms and resilience, making it difficult to effectively manage symptoms and navigate daily challenges.

5. Emotional Wellbeing:

The emotional impact of living with a chronic illness can be profound, leading to feelings of depression, anxiety, grief, or isolation. Stressful life events, medical appointments, and functional limitations associated with EDS may exacerbate emotional distress and impact overall quality of life.

Understanding the interconnectedness of stress and EDS symptoms underscores the importance of adopting proactive strategies to manage stress and promote emotional wellbeing. By recognizing stress triggers, cultivating healthy coping mechanisms, and fostering resilience, individuals with EDS can mitigate the impact of stress on their symptoms and enhance their overall quality of life.

8.2 Developing Stress-Management Techniques: Relaxation, Mindfulness, and Meditation

Effectively managing stress is essential for individuals with Ehlers-Danlos Syndrome (EDS) to minimize symptom exacerbation, improve overall wellbeing, and enhance resilience in the face of life's challenges. Incorporating relaxation, mindfulness, and meditation techniques into daily life can help individuals cope with stress more effectively. Here are some stress-management techniques tailored for individuals with EDS:

1. Deep Breathing Exercises:

Deep breathing exercises, such as diaphragmatic breathing or paced breathing, promote relaxation and activate the body's natural relaxation response. Encourage individuals to practice deep breathing techniques regularly to reduce muscle tension, calm the nervous system, and enhance oxygenation.

2. Progressive Muscle Relaxation (PMR):

Progressive muscle relaxation involves systematically tensing and relaxing muscle groups throughout the body to release tension and promote physical and mental relaxation. Guided PMR exercises can help individuals with EDS become more aware of muscle tension patterns and learn to release tension consciously.

3. Mindfulness Meditation:

Mindfulness meditation involves cultivating present-moment awareness and nonjudgmental acceptance of thoughts, feelings, and sensations. Mindfulness-based practices, such as body scans, mindful breathing, or loving-kindness meditation, can help individuals with EDS develop resilience, reduce stress reactivity, and improve emotional regulation.

4. Guided Imagery and Visualization:

Guided imagery and visualization techniques involve mentally picturing peaceful scenes, positive outcomes, or healing processes to evoke relaxation and positive emotions. Guided imagery scripts or recordings tailored to individual preferences can serve as powerful tools for managing stress and promoting inner peace.

5. Yoga and Tai Chi:

Yoga and Tai Chi are mind-body practices that integrate gentle movements, breathwork, and mindfulness techniques to improve physical strength, flexibility, and relaxation. Modified yoga poses and Tai Chi exercises adapted for individuals with EDS can provide gentle exercise, stress relief, and emotional balance.

6. Creative Expression:

Engaging in creative activities such as art therapy, music therapy, journaling, or expressive writing can serve as outlets for self-expression, emotional processing, and stress relief. Encourage individuals to explore creative hobbies that resonate with their interests and preferences to foster self-awareness and relaxation.

7. Nature Therapy:

Spending time in nature, known as nature therapy or ecotherapy, can promote relaxation, reduce stress, and enhance overall wellbeing. Encourage individuals to connect with the natural world through activities such as walking in nature, gardening, birdwatching, or simply enjoying outdoor environments.

8. Social Support and Connection:

Maintaining social connections and seeking support from friends, family members, support groups, or mental health professionals can provide valuable emotional support and validation. Connecting with others who understand the challenges of living with EDS can reduce feelings of isolation and promote a sense of belonging and resilience.

By incorporating these stress-management techniques into daily life, individuals with Ehlers-Danlos Syndrome (EDS) can cultivate a greater sense of calm, balance, and emotional resilience, allowing them to navigate the ups and downs of life with greater ease and grace.

8.3 Building Emotional Resilience: Strategies for Coping with Challenges

Emotional resilience is the ability to adapt and bounce back from adversity, setbacks, and stressors, and it plays a crucial role in coping with the challenges of living with Ehlers-Danlos Syndrome (EDS). Building emotional resilience involves developing skills, attitudes, and strategies to effectively manage stress, navigate difficulties, and maintain a positive outlook. Here are some strategies for building emotional resilience tailored for individuals with EDS:

1. Cultivate Self-Compassion:

Practice self-compassion by treating yourself with kindness, understanding, and acceptance, especially during times of pain, fatigue, or frustration. Acknowledge your struggles and limitations without self-judgment, and offer yourself the same compassion and support you would offer to a loved one.

2. Foster Positive Relationships:

Nurture supportive relationships with friends, family members, healthcare providers, and fellow individuals with EDS who understand and validate your experiences. Surround yourself with people who uplift and empower you, and seek out social connections that foster a sense of belonging and understanding.

3. Develop Adaptive Coping Strategies:

Identify and cultivate adaptive coping strategies that help you effectively manage stress and cope with the challenges of living with EDS. Experiment with different coping techniques, such as problem-solving, reframing negative thoughts, seeking social support, or engaging in enjoyable activities, to discover what works best for you.

4. Practice Emotional Regulation:

Learn to recognize and regulate your emotions in healthy and constructive ways. Practice mindfulness techniques, such as deep breathing or grounding exercises, to calm the nervous system and reduce emotional reactivity. Allow yourself to experience and express emotions without judgment, and seek outlets for emotional expression and processing.

5. Find Meaning and Purpose:

Explore activities, interests, or values that give your life meaning and purpose, and actively engage in pursuits that align with your passions and aspirations. Cultivate a sense of purpose by contributing to causes you care about, pursuing creative endeavors, or volunteering in your community, fostering a sense of fulfillment and connection.

6. Build Adaptive Thinking Patterns:

Challenge and reframe negative thinking patterns that contribute to feelings of hopelessness, helplessness, or despair. Practice cognitive restructuring techniques to replace unhelpful thoughts with more balanced and realistic perspectives, emphasizing strengths, resources, and opportunities for growth.

7. Set Realistic Goals:

Set realistic and achievable goals that reflect your values, priorities, and capabilities, taking into account the fluctuations and unpredictability of EDS symptoms. Break larger goals into smaller, manageable steps, and celebrate progress and accomplishments along the way, fostering a sense of accomplishment and self-efficacy.

8. Practice Resilience-Building Activities:

Engage in resilience-building activities that promote physical, emotional, and spiritual wellbeing, such as regular exercise, mindfulness meditation, creative expression, gratitude practice, or spending time in nature. Cultivate habits and routines that support resilience and self-care, nurturing your mind, body, and spirit.

By implementing these strategies for building emotional resilience, individuals with Ehlers-Danlos Syndrome (EDS) can strengthen their capacity to cope with adversity, thrive in the face of challenges, and cultivate a greater sense of inner strength, hope, and optimism in their journey toward wellness and wellbeing.

HEALTHY SLEEP HABITS

with Ehlers-Danlos Syndrome EDS

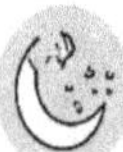

Create a consistent sleep a wag dieey schedule

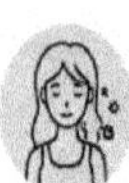

Estabish you bedtime routine

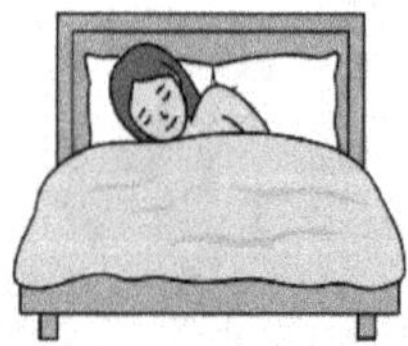

Establisy sleep environment for comfort for comfort and support

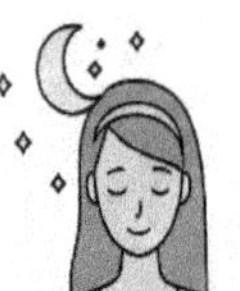

Practice stress reatecia thanpane ant muscle gentle stretching adodes.

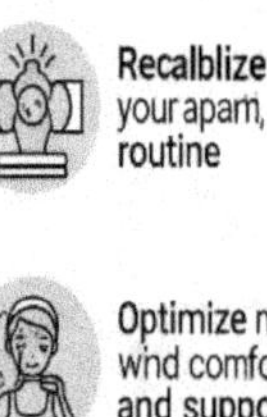

Recalblize bee sleep your aparn, and routine

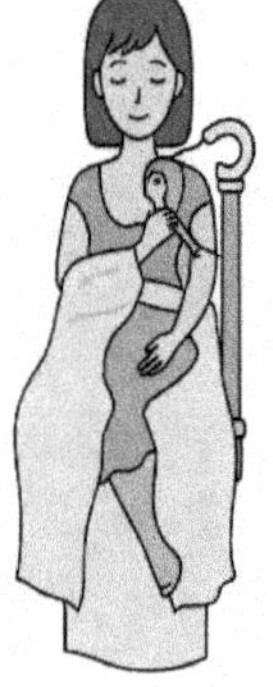

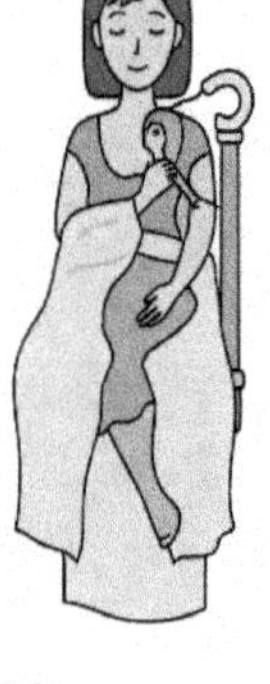

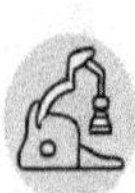

Optimize management wind comfort die and support

Stectice management with chelcus dous greccile.

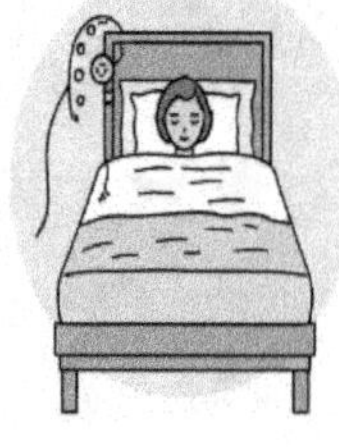

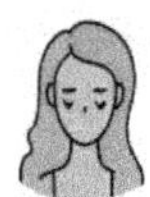

Joint pain snerle fatiguer

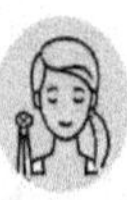

Sleep-reated breathing disorters

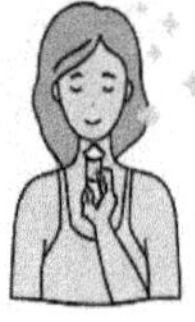

Mindfulesss, triso fatigue honmed gentle stretching

Ondipacl ant inaragement sceap ho uold ond soinse and tre geunole.

CHAPTER NINE

FINDING YOUR VOICE: COMMUNICATION AND ADVOCACY WITH EDS

9.1 Effective Communication with Doctors and Healthcare Providers

Establishing clear and productive communication with doctors and healthcare providers is essential for individuals with Ehlers-Danlos Syndrome (EDS) to receive optimal care and support. Effective communication involves actively engaging with healthcare professionals, advocating for your needs, and fostering collaborative relationships. Here are some strategies for effective communication:

1. Prepare for Appointments:

Before appointments, take time to prepare a list of symptoms, questions, and concerns to discuss with your healthcare provider. Bring along relevant medical records, test results, and a medication list to provide comprehensive information about your health status.

2. Be Honest and Transparent:

Be open and honest about your symptoms, experiences, and treatment preferences during appointments. Share any changes in symptoms or medication side effects, and don't hesitate to ask questions or seek clarification about your condition and treatment options.

3. Use Clear and Specific Language:

Communicate clearly and concisely using simple language to ensure mutual understanding between you and your healthcare provider. Avoid medical jargon or terminology that may be unfamiliar, and ask for explanations or definitions if needed to clarify information.

4. Actively Participate in Decision-Making:

Engage in shared decision-making with your healthcare provider by expressing your preferences, values, and goals regarding treatment options. Collaboratively discuss the benefits, risks, and alternatives of different interventions to make informed decisions that align with your needs and priorities.

5. Advocate for Comprehensive Care:

Advocate for comprehensive care by addressing the multidimensional aspects of EDS, including physical, emotional, and social factors. Emphasize the importance of holistic care that considers all aspects of your health and wellbeing, and advocate for referrals to specialists or allied health professionals as needed.

6. Seek Second Opinions if Necessary:

If you have concerns about your diagnosis or treatment plan, don't hesitate to seek a second opinion from another healthcare provider or specialist with expertise in EDS. Obtaining additional perspectives can offer valuable insights and help you make well-informed decisions about your care.

7. Follow Up and Stay Engaged:

Follow up with your healthcare provider regularly to monitor your progress, discuss treatment efficacy, and address any ongoing concerns or new symptoms. Stay engaged in your healthcare by actively participating in follow-up appointments, adhering to treatment recommendations, and advocating for adjustments as needed.

By adopting these strategies for effective communication with doctors and healthcare providers, individuals with Ehlers-Danlos Syndrome (EDS) can enhance their healthcare experiences, improve treatment outcomes, and empower themselves as active participants in their care journey.

9.2 Advocating for Your Needs: Empowering Yourself in Medical Settings

Advocating for your needs in medical settings is crucial for individuals with Ehlers-Danlos Syndrome (EDS) to ensure that their concerns are heard, their preferences are respected, and their care is tailored to their unique needs. Empowering yourself as a self-advocate involves assertively expressing your needs, rights, and boundaries while collaborating with healthcare professionals. Here are some strategies for advocating for your needs:

1. Educate Yourself:

Take the time to educate yourself about Ehlers-Danlos Syndrome (EDS), including its symptoms, potential complications, treatment options, and self-care strategies. Knowledge empowers you to make informed decisions about your health and effectively communicate with healthcare providers.

2. Know Your Rights:

Familiarize yourself with your rights as a patient, including the right to informed consent, confidentiality, respectful treatment, and access to your medical records. Advocate for your rights by speaking up if you feel they are being violated or if you have concerns about the quality of care you're receiving.

3. Communicate Assertively:

Assertively communicate your needs, concerns, and boundaries with healthcare providers in a clear, respectful, and confident manner. Use "I" statements to express how you're feeling and what you need, and don't hesitate to advocate for accommodations or modifications that support your wellbeing.

4. Bring a Support Person:

Consider bringing a trusted friend, family member, or advocate to medical appointments for support and assistance in advocating for your needs. A supportive companion can help you remember important information, ask questions, and provide emotional support during challenging discussions.

5. Keep a Health Journal:

Maintain a health journal or diary to document your symptoms, medication side effects, appointments, and any changes in your health status. Keeping detailed records can help you track patterns, identify triggers, and provide valuable information to healthcare providers for more accurate diagnosis and treatment.

6. Seek Referrals to Specialists:

If you require specialized care or treatment for specific EDS-related issues, advocate for referrals to specialists with expertise in connective tissue disorders, such as geneticists, rheumatologists, orthopedic surgeons, or pain management specialists. Collaborating with specialists can ensure comprehensive and personalized care.

7. Stay Persistent and Resilient:

Be persistent in advocating for your needs, even if you encounter challenges or setbacks along the way. Don't be discouraged by dismissive attitudes or lack of understanding from healthcare providers; continue to assert your needs and seek out supportive professionals who are willing to partner with you in your care.

Empowering yourself as a self-advocate requires courage, resilience, and determination, but it can lead to improved healthcare experiences, enhanced treatment outcomes, and a greater sense of control over your health and wellbeing.

9.3 Building a Strong Support System: Enlisting the Help of Family and Friends

Building a strong support system is essential for individuals with Ehlers-Danlos Syndrome (EDS) to navigate the challenges of living with a chronic illness, access emotional support, and receive practical assistance when needed. Enlisting the help of family and friends can provide invaluable social, emotional, and practical support, fostering resilience and wellbeing. Here are some strategies for building a strong support system:

1. Foster Open Communication:

Create an environment of open communication with your family and friends, where you feel comfortable expressing your needs, concerns, and emotions related to EDS. Encourage honest dialogue, active listening, and mutual understanding to strengthen your relationships and support network.

2. Educate Loved Ones about EDS:

Educate your family and friends about Ehlers-Danlos Syndrome (EDS), including its symptoms, treatment options, and the impact it has on your daily life. Help them understand the challenges you face and the support you need to manage your condition effectively.

3. Clarify Support Needs:

Clearly communicate your support needs and preferences to your loved ones, including practical assistance with daily tasks, emotional support during difficult times, or simply having someone to talk to when you're feeling overwhelmed. Be specific about how they can help and what would be most beneficial for you.

4. Set Realistic Expectations:

Set realistic expectations for yourself and your loved ones regarding what you can reasonably manage and accomplish while living with EDS. Be honest about your limitations and boundaries, and encourage open dialogue about how you can work together to navigate challenges and find solutions.

5. Cultivate Empathy and Understanding:

Cultivate empathy and understanding among your family and friends by encouraging them to put themselves in your shoes and consider the impact of EDS on your life. Foster a supportive and compassionate environment where you feel validated, accepted, and valued for who you are beyond your illness.

6. Seek Peer Support:

Connect with other individuals with EDS and their caregivers through support groups, online forums, or community organizations to share experiences, exchange advice, and find solidarity in your journey. Peer support can provide a unique source of empathy, validation, and encouragement from those who truly understand what you're going through.

7. Express Gratitude and Appreciation:

Express gratitude and appreciation to your family and friends for their support, kindness, and understanding as you navigate life with EDS. Acknowledge the contributions they make to your wellbeing, and let them know how much their presence and assistance mean to you.

By actively building and nurturing a strong support system of family and friends, individuals with Ehlers-Danlos Syndrome (EDS) can cultivate resilience, foster wellbeing, and enhance their quality of life despite the challenges posed by their condition.

TREATMENT
EHLERS-DANLOS SYNDROME

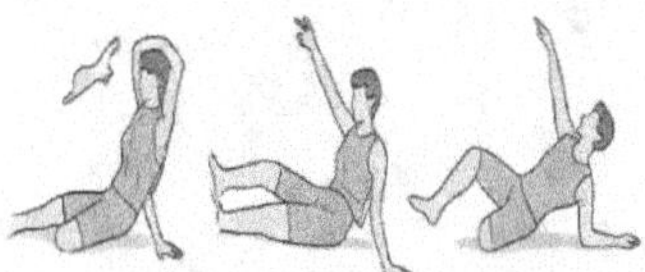
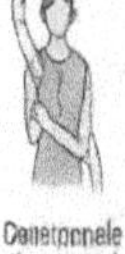
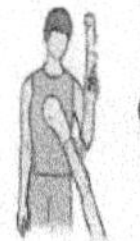
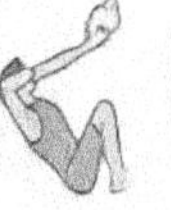
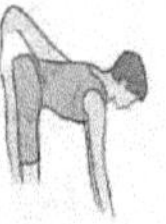

Physical Therapy

Stretchs

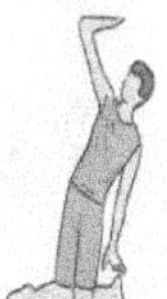
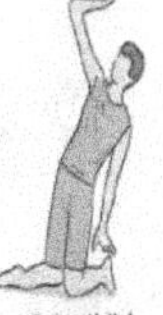

Barenels Mobilization exereiens

Joint stbiki areed toneor ahrereiens

Hniris eiugrane Mociirpans a ciort and simertun

PHYSICAL THERAPY

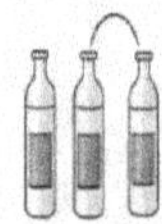
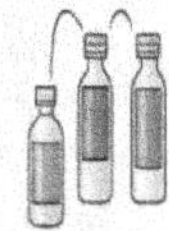
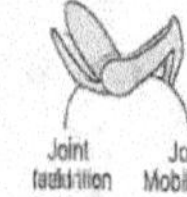

MEINTX-MEDICATIONS

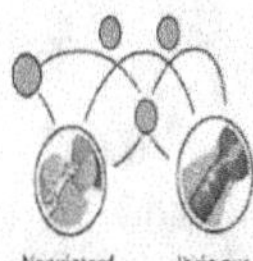

PHYSICAL THERAMPS

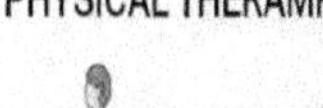
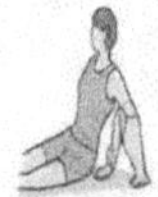
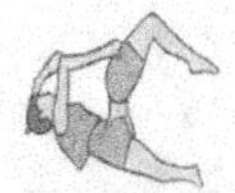
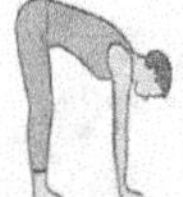

Vioin isarneley ther eun ial exerciens

Thementina seiort isen anpation trioid mobliiaton

Hove of eeint ihreshome ahraty liendons pretepeius

SURGICAL INTERVNTIONS

SURGICAL INTERVNTIONS

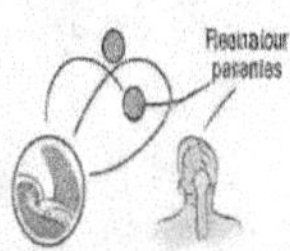
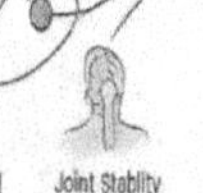
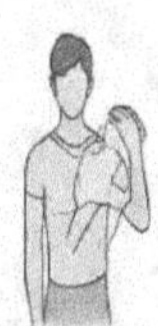
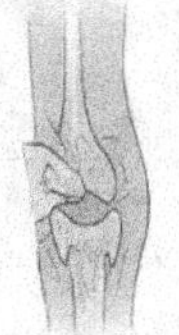
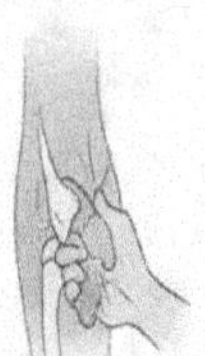
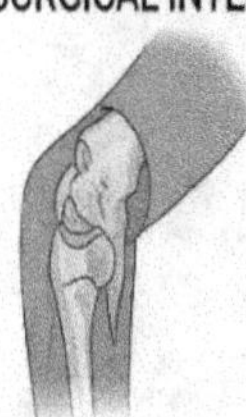
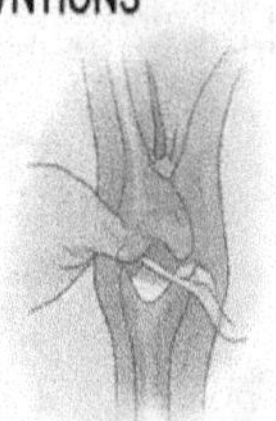

Ehlers-Danloc ines Joint sunhets of beresdars

Pleck a witgrinuntters eeckaerrr anel iomaiiore yous

Fletenn pranlroaloal blnd tooirador oairt s iegel

Ehlers-Dies hotesebhos to mepieliliget and ligerments uaht thement.

Ehlers-Danlo Froertuetend Belertrone. Thie soptoon et clseligenbertertiepart.

TREATMENT
EHLERS-DANLOS SYNDROME

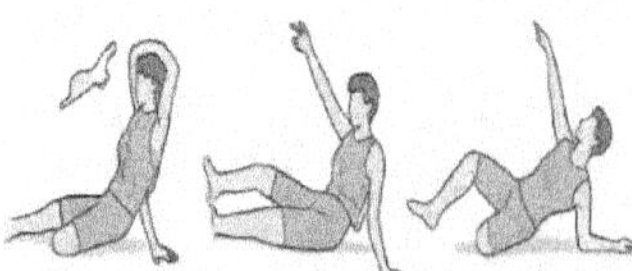
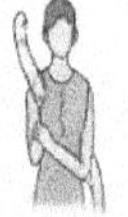
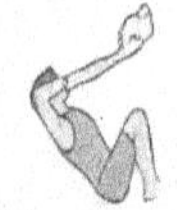
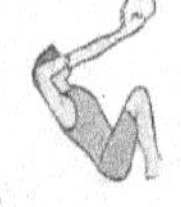
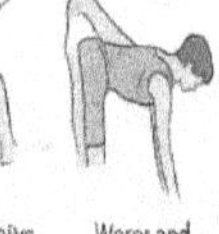

PHYSICAL THERAPY

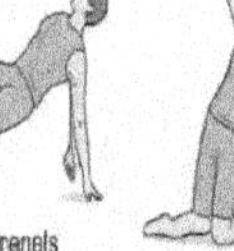
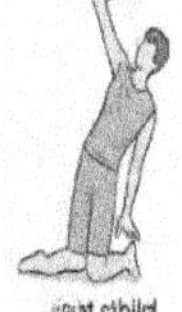
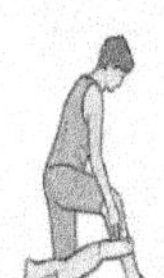
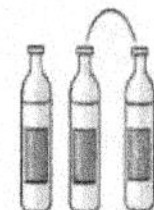

PHYSICAL THERAMPS

MEINTX-MEDICATIONS

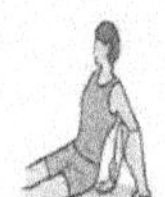
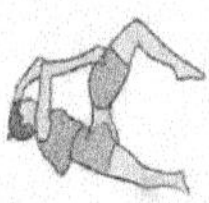
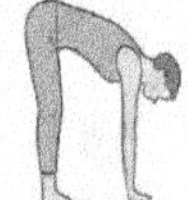
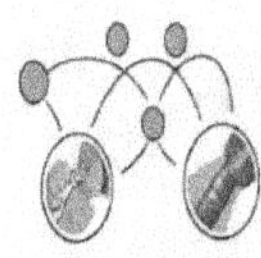
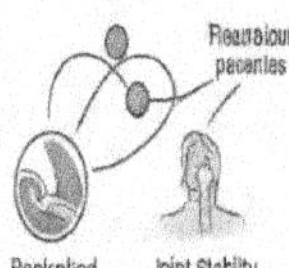

SURGICAL INTERVNTIONS

SURGICAL INTERVNTIONS

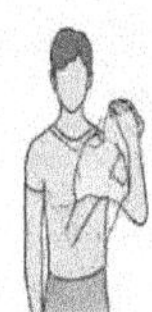
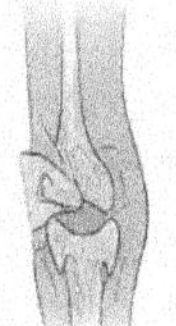
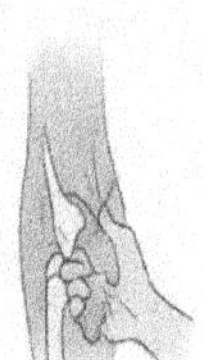
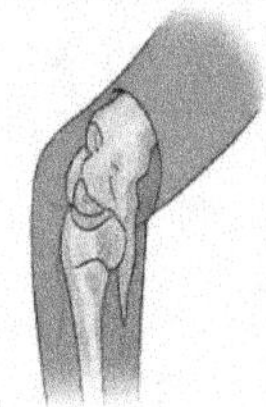
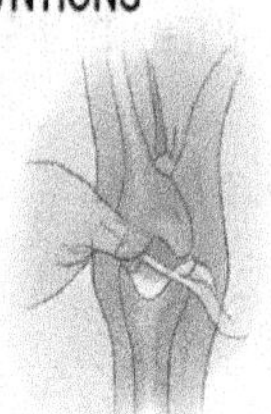

CHAPTER TEN

CREATING A SAFE AND SUPPORTIVE ENVIRONMENT

10.1 Adapting Your Home for Optimal Living with EDS

Adapting your home environment to accommodate the unique needs of Ehlers-Danlos Syndrome (EDS) can significantly enhance your comfort, safety, and quality of life. Making modifications and adjustments to your living space can help minimize physical strain, reduce the risk of injuries, and promote independence. Here are some strategies for adapting your home for optimal living with EDS:

1. Create Accessibility:

Ensure that your home is accessible and navigable, especially if you experience mobility challenges or use assistive devices. Remove clutter, obstacles, and tripping hazards from walkways and pathways to facilitate safe movement throughout your home.

2. Install Handrails and Grab Bars:

Install handrails and grab bars in key areas of your home, such as staircases, bathrooms, and hallways, to provide additional support and stability. Securely mount these fixtures to walls to assist with balance, mobility, and transferring between surfaces.

3. Modify Furniture:

Choose furniture with ergonomic designs and features that provide adequate support and comfort for individuals with EDS. opt for chairs, sofas, and beds with adjustable height, lumbar support, and cushioning to minimize strain on joints and muscles.

4. Improve Lighting:

Enhance lighting in your home to reduce the risk of falls and improve visibility, especially in dimly lit areas or during nighttime. Use a combination of natural and artificial lighting sources, including overhead lights, task lighting, and floor lamps, to create a well-lit and safe environment.

5. Organize and Declutter:

Organize your home environment to minimize the need for excessive bending, reaching, or lifting. Use storage solutions such as shelves, cabinets, and drawers to keep frequently used items within easy reach and maintain a clutter-free living space.

6. Create Rest Zones:

Designate specific areas in your home as rest zones where you can relax, unwind, and recharge. Consider incorporating comfortable seating, supportive pillows, and calming décor elements to promote relaxation and alleviate stress on your body.

7. Install Safety Features:

Install safety features such as smoke detectors, carbon monoxide detectors, and emergency alert systems to ensure your home is equipped to handle unforeseen emergencies. Regularly check and maintain these safety devices to ensure they are functioning properly.

8. Seek Professional Assistance:

Consult with occupational therapists, home modification specialists, or accessibility experts for personalized recommendations and guidance on adapting your home to better suit your needs. These professionals can assess your home environment and recommend modifications tailored to your specific requirements.

By adapting your home environment to accommodate the challenges of living with EDS, you can create a safe, supportive, and comfortable living space that promotes independence, mobility, and overall wellbeing.

10.2 Assistive Devices and Tools for Daily Activities

Assistive devices and tools play a crucial role in enhancing independence, mobility, and functionality for individuals with Ehlers-Danlos Syndrome (EDS). These specialized devices are designed to compensate for physical limitations, reduce strain on joints and muscles, and facilitate daily activities and tasks. Here are some common assistive devices and tools that can benefit individuals with EDS:

1. Mobility Aids:

Mobility aids such as canes, walkers, crutches, and wheelchairs provide support and stability for individuals with EDS who experience difficulties with balance, walking, or standing for extended periods. Choose the appropriate mobility aid based on your specific needs and mobility level.

2. Orthopedic Braces and Supports:

Orthopedic braces, splints, and supports help stabilize and protect joints affected by hypermobility, instability, or subluxations commonly associated with EDS. These devices provide external support, alignment, and proprioceptive feedback to reduce pain and enhance joint function.

3. Adaptive Kitchen Tools:

Adaptive kitchen tools and utensils with ergonomic designs and specialized features make meal preparation and cooking tasks more manageable for individuals with EDS. Look for tools such as easy-grip handles, jar openers, adaptive cutting boards, and utensils with built-in stability aids.

4. Bathroom Safety Equipment:

Bathroom safety equipment such as shower chairs, transfer benches, grab bars, and raised toilet seats promote safety and independence for individuals with EDS when performing personal hygiene tasks. Install these devices to prevent slips, falls, and injuries in wet or slippery environments.

5. Ergonomic Furniture:

Ergonomic furniture designed for comfort and support can help alleviate musculoskeletal strain and discomfort associated with prolonged sitting or lying down. Invest in ergonomic chairs, adjustable desks, supportive mattresses, and pillows to maintain proper posture and reduce pressure on sensitive areas.

6. Adaptive Dressing Aids:

Adaptive dressing aids such as button hooks, zipper pulls, dressing sticks, and elastic shoelaces simplify the process of getting dressed and undressed for individuals with EDS who experience joint hypermobility or dexterity challenges. These aids promote independence and autonomy in daily dressing routines.

7. Environmental Modifications:

Make modifications to your home environment, such as installing handrails, ramps, stairlifts, and accessible doorways, to improve accessibility and facilitate independent living for individuals with EDS. Customize your living space to accommodate mobility aids and assistive devices effectively.

8. Communication and Writing Aids:

Communication and writing aids such as voice-to-text software, ergonomic keyboards, adaptive pens, and page turners assist individuals with EDS who experience hand weakness, pain, or limited mobility in performing writing or typing tasks. These aids enable effective communication and participation in daily activities.

By incorporating assistive devices and tools into daily routines, individuals with Ehlers-Danlos Syndrome (EDS) can overcome physical challenges, maintain independence, and improve their overall quality of life.

Pacing and energy conservation strategies are essential for individuals with Ehlers-Danlos Syndrome (EDS) to manage fatigue, prevent overexertion, and optimize energy levels throughout the day. By pacing activities, prioritizing rest, and balancing periods of exertion with periods of recovery, individuals with EDS can minimize symptom exacerbation and enhance their overall wellbeing. Here are some effective strategies for pacing and energy conservation:

1. Listen to Your Body:

Pay attention to your body's signals and cues, including pain, fatigue, and discomfort, to gauge your energy levels and determine when to rest or modify activities. Be mindful of early warning signs of overexertion and adjust your pace accordingly to avoid pushing beyond your limits.

2. Prioritize Activities:

Prioritize essential tasks and activities based on their importance and urgency, focusing on accomplishing high-priority tasks during periods of higher energy and postponing non-essential activities for times when you feel more rested and capable.

3. Break Tasks into Manageable Segments:

Break down larger tasks or projects into smaller, more manageable segments to avoid overwhelming yourself and conserve energy. Pace yourself by alternating between periods of activity and rest, taking short breaks to rest and recharge as needed.

4. Use Energy-Saving Techniques:

Implement energy-saving techniques such as using assistive devices, planning efficient movement patterns, and delegating tasks to conserve energy and minimize physical strain. Use adaptive strategies and tools to streamline activities and reduce unnecessary exertion.

5. Practice Restorative Activities:

Incorporate restorative activities such as relaxation techniques, mindfulness practices, gentle stretching, and deep breathing exercises into your daily routine to promote relaxation, reduce stress, and replenish energy reserves. Schedule regular periods of rest and relaxation throughout the day to prevent fatigue accumulation.

6. Set Realistic Goals:

Set realistic goals and expectations for yourself, considering your current capabilities, limitations, and energy levels. Break goals down into achievable steps and celebrate progress, however small, to maintain motivation and momentum.

7. Establish Boundaries:

Establish boundaries with yourself and others to protect your energy and avoid overcommitting to activities or obligations that may drain your resources. Learn to say no when necessary and prioritize self-care to maintain balance and prevent burnout.

8. Monitor and Adjust:

Regularly monitor your energy levels, symptoms, and activity levels to assess how well pacing and energy conservation strategies are working for you. Be flexible and willing to adjust your approach as needed based on changes in your health, circumstances, or priorities.

By adopting pacing and energy conservation techniques, individuals with Ehlers-Danlos Syndrome (EDS) can effectively manage their energy levels, reduce symptom exacerbation, and improve their overall quality of life.

HEALTHY SLEEP HABITS

with Ehlers-Danlos Syndrome EDS

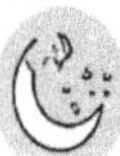

Create a consistant sleep a way duiey schedule

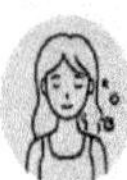

Estabish you bedtime routine

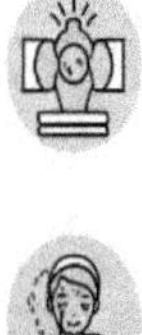

Recalblize bee sleep your aparn, and routine

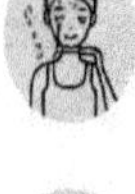

Optimize management wind comfort die and support

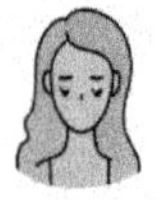

Stectice management with xcleus dous greccile.

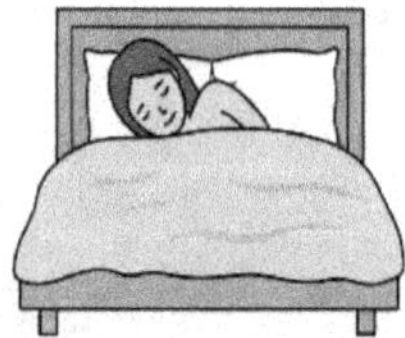

Establisy sleep environment for comfort for comfort and support

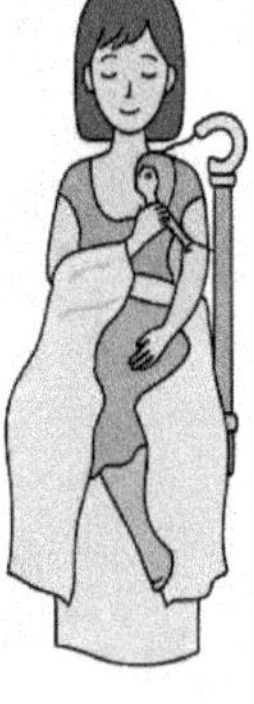

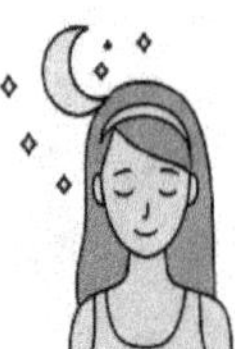

Seop st criarty sleep peep mucles stedoles.

Practice stress reatecta thanpane ant muscle gentle stretching adodes.

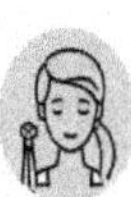

Joint pain snerle fatiguer

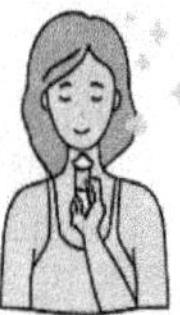

Sleep-reated breathing disorters

Mindfulesss, triiso fatigue honmed gentle stretching

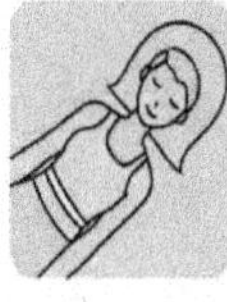

Ondi pacl ant inaragement sceap ho uold ond soinse and tre geunole.

CHAPTER ELEVEN

LIVING A FULFILLING LIFE: RELATIONSHIPS, WORK, AND PLAY

11.1 Maintaining Healthy Relationships: Setting Boundaries and Advocating for Your Needs

Maintaining healthy relationships is essential for individuals with Ehlers-Danlos Syndrome (EDS) to cultivate a supportive network and navigate the challenges of living with a chronic condition. Setting boundaries and advocating for your needs are crucial aspects of nurturing positive relationships that respect your physical and emotional wellbeing. Here are some strategies for maintaining healthy relationships with family, friends, and loved ones:

1. Open Communication:

Establish open and honest communication with your loved ones about your condition, symptoms, and limitations. Share information about EDS and how it affects your daily life to foster understanding, empathy, and support.

2. Set Clear Boundaries:

Set clear boundaries with others regarding your physical capabilities, energy levels, and need for rest and self-care. Communicate your boundaries assertively and respectfully, and advocate for your needs without feeling guilty or ashamed.

3. Prioritize Self-Care:

Prioritize self-care and prioritize activities that promote your health and wellbeing. Communicate your self-care needs to your loved ones and seek their understanding and cooperation in respecting your boundaries and limitations.

4. Practice Assertiveness:

Practice assertiveness techniques to express your needs, preferences, and limitations assertively and confidently. Use "I" statements to communicate your feelings and avoid blaming or criticizing others for their actions or behaviors.

5. Seek Support:

Seek support from trusted friends, family members, or support groups who understand your challenges and can offer empathy, encouragement, and practical assistance when needed. Surround yourself with individuals who uplift and validate your experiences.

6. Foster Mutual Respect:

Foster mutual respect and understanding in your relationships by actively listening to others, validating their feelings, and acknowledging their perspectives. Cultivate empathy, compassion, and patience in your interactions with loved ones.

7. Set Realistic Expectations:

Set realistic expectations for yourself and others, recognizing that living with EDS may require adjustments and accommodations. Be flexible and adaptable in your relationships, and avoid comparing yourself to others or feeling pressured to meet unrealistic standards.

8. Practice Self-Compassion:

Practice self-compassion and self-acceptance as you navigate the ups and downs of living with EDS. Be kind and patient with yourself, and recognize your strengths, resilience, and inherent worth as a person.

By setting boundaries, advocating for your needs, and fostering healthy communication and mutual respect in your relationships, you can cultivate a supportive network of friends and family who empower and uplift you on your journey with EDS.

11.2 Finding Meaningful Work: Career Options and Considerations for People with EDS

Finding meaningful work and pursuing a fulfilling career is possible for individuals with Ehlers-Danlos Syndrome (EDS), although it may require careful consideration, accommodations, and flexibility to accommodate the challenges associated with the condition. Here are some career options and considerations for people with EDS:

1. Flexible Work Arrangements:

Explore flexible work arrangements such as telecommuting, part-time employment, freelance work, or self-employment to accommodate fluctuations in symptoms and energy levels. Look for opportunities that allow you to work from home or customize your schedule to better manage your condition.

2. Disability Employment Services:

Consider accessing disability employment services or vocational rehabilitation programs that provide support, resources, and assistance with job placement, accommodations, and career development for individuals with disabilities, including EDS.

3. Remote or Desk-Based Jobs:

Consider pursuing remote or desk-based jobs that require minimal physical exertion and offer opportunities for sedentary work, such as administrative roles, customer service positions, writing and editing, graphic design, programming, or data entry.

4. Career Counseling:

Seek guidance from career counselors or vocational specialists who can help you explore your interests, skills, and strengths, and identify suitable career paths and job opportunities that align with your abilities and limitations.

5. Advocacy and Education:

Consider pursuing careers in advocacy, education, healthcare, or social services where you can use your personal experiences with EDS to raise awareness, support others, and drive positive change in your community or profession.

6. Accommodations and Modifications:

Request accommodations and modifications in the workplace to address specific challenges related to EDS, such as ergonomic furniture, assistive technology, flexible scheduling, or modified job duties. Advocate for your needs and rights under the Americans with Disabilities Act (ADA) or similar legislation.

7. Self-Employment and Entrepreneurship:

Explore self-employment and entrepreneurship opportunities that allow you to create your own schedule, control your workload, and tailor your business activities to accommodate your health needs and preferences.

8. Pursue Your Passions:

Identify and pursue career paths that align with your passions, interests, and values, and bring you a sense of fulfillment, purpose, and joy. Don't let EDS define or limit your career aspirations—focus on your strengths and abilities, and find ways to thrive in your chosen field.

By exploring diverse career options, seeking accommodations and support when needed, and prioritizing your health and wellbeing, you can find meaningful work and build a successful career that aligns with your abilities and aspirations despite the challenges of living with EDS.

Engaging in leisure activities and socialization is essential for promoting mental and emotional wellbeing and enhancing quality of life for individuals with Ehlers-Danlos Syndrome (EDS). Despite the challenges posed by the condition, there are various leisure activities and social opportunities that you can explore to find joy, fulfillment, and connection. Here are some suggestions for finding activities you enjoy and staying connected:

1. Pursue Low-Impact Hobbies:

Explore hobbies and leisure activities that are low-impact and gentle on your body, such as painting, drawing, crafting, gardening, photography, writing, reading, or listening to music. Choose activities that you find enjoyable, relaxing, and fulfilling, and adapt them to accommodate your energy levels and physical abilities.

2. Participate in Support Groups:

Join local or online support groups for individuals with EDS or chronic illnesses where you can connect with others who understand your experiences, share tips and resources, and offer mutual support and encouragement. Engage in group discussions, attend meetings or events, and build meaningful relationships with fellow members.

3. Attend Social Events:

Attend social events, gatherings, or meetups in your community that cater to your interests and passions, such as art classes, book clubs, support group meetings, or wellness workshops. Look for inclusive and accessible venues and activities that accommodate your needs and preferences.

4. Volunteer Opportunities:

Explore volunteer opportunities with organizations or causes that are meaningful to you and align with your values and interests. Volunteer work can provide a sense of purpose, social connection, and fulfillment, while also allowing you to contribute to positive change in your community.

5. Stay Connected Virtually:

Stay connected with friends, family, and loved ones through virtual means such as video calls, social media, online forums, or virtual game nights. Use technology to bridge geographical distances and maintain relationships with those who are unable to meet in person.

6. Practice Self-Care Outings:

Plan self-care outings or excursions that allow you to enjoy leisure activities while prioritizing your health and wellbeing. Take leisurely walks in nature, visit museums or art galleries, attend gentle yoga or meditation classes, or treat yourself to a relaxing spa day.

7. Explore Adaptive Sports and Recreation:

Explore adaptive sports and recreational activities that are suitable for individuals with varying abilities and mobility levels, such as adaptive yoga, wheelchair basketball, swimming, or seated aerobics. Participate in adaptive sports programs or classes tailored to accommodate your specific needs and preferences.

8. Foster Meaningful Connections:

Foster meaningful connections and relationships with others by being authentic, vulnerable, and compassionate in your interactions. Be open to making new friends, sharing your experiences, and supporting others on their journey, both within the EDS community and beyond.

By actively engaging in leisure activities, socializing with others, and fostering meaningful connections and relationships, individuals with EDS can enrich their lives, cultivate a sense of belonging, and experience joy, fulfillment, and camaraderie despite the challenges posed by the condition.

HEALTHY SLEEP HABITS

with Ehlers-Danlos Syndrome EDS

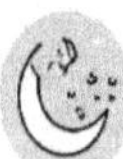

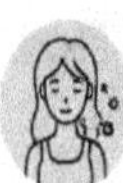

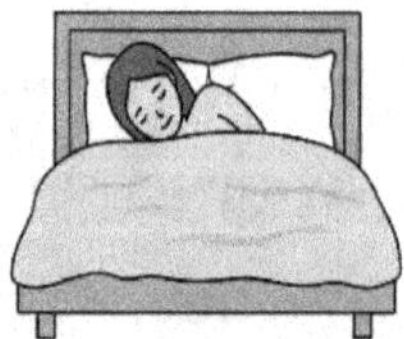

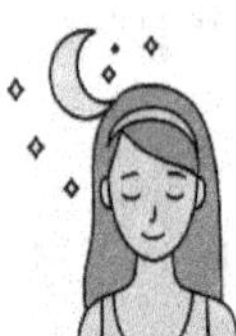

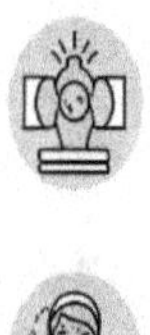

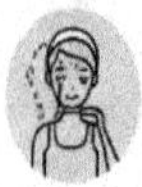

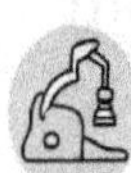

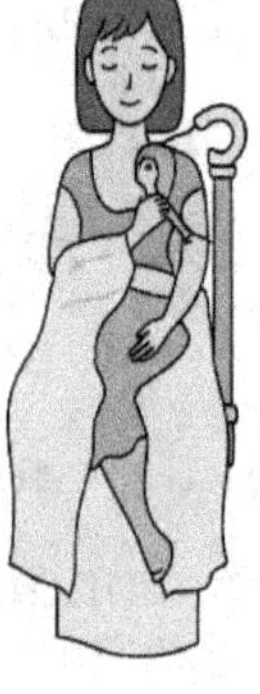

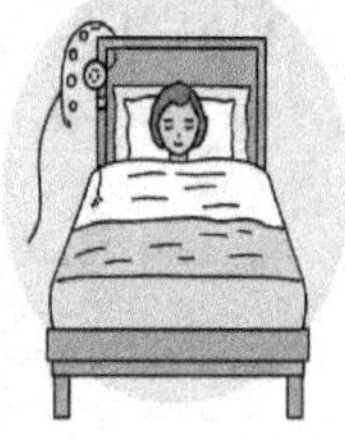

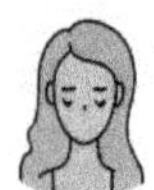

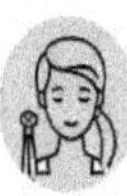

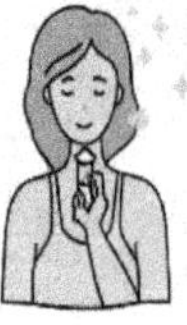

CHAPTER TWELVE

A LOOK TO THE FUTURE: LIVING WITH HOPE AND OPTIMISM

12.1 The Future of EDS Research and Treatment: Staying Up-to-Date on Advancements

Ehlers-Danlos Syndrome (EDS) research and treatment are constantly evolving, driven by ongoing scientific discoveries and advancements in medical technology. Staying informed about these developments is crucial for individuals with EDS and their caregivers. Here's how to stay up-to-date and what to expect in the future of EDS research and treatment:

1. Follow Research Publications:

Regularly read research publications and journals that focus on genetic disorders, connective tissue diseases, and specifically EDS. Websites like PubMed and Google Scholar can provide access to the latest studies and clinical trials.

2. Engage with EDS Organizations:

Engage with organizations such as the Ehlers-Danlos Society, which provides updates on research, treatment options, and advocacy efforts. These organizations often host conferences, webinars, and workshops that disseminate cutting-edge information.

3. Participate in Clinical Trials:

Consider participating in clinical trials that focus on EDS. Clinical trials are essential for developing new treatments and understanding the condition better. Websites like ClinicalTrials.gov list ongoing studies you might qualify for.

4. Genetic Research and Testing:

Advances in genetic research and testing are shedding light on the molecular basis of EDS. New genetic testing methods can help in identifying specific mutations, leading to more accurate diagnoses and personalized treatment plans.

5. Novel Therapeutics:

Keep an eye on emerging therapies and treatments, such as gene therapy, biologics, and novel pharmacological interventions. These advancements hold promise for addressing the root causes of EDS and managing symptoms more effectively.

6. Multidisciplinary Care Models:

Multidisciplinary care models that involve coordinated care from various specialists (geneticists, rheumatologists, physiotherapists, etc.) are becoming more common. This approach ensures comprehensive care that addresses the diverse manifestations of EDS.

7. Patient Registries and Big Data:

Patient registries and big data analytics are playing a significant role in understanding EDS on a larger scale. By contributing to these registries, patients can help researchers identify trends, treatment outcomes, and potential new therapeutic targets.

8. Advocacy for Research Funding:

Advocate for increased funding for EDS research by supporting organizations and participating in awareness campaigns. Greater funding can accelerate the pace of research and lead to breakthroughs in understanding and treating EDS.

By staying informed and engaged with the latest research and treatment advancements, individuals with EDS can benefit from new developments and contribute to the collective knowledge and understanding of the condition.

12.2 Embracing a Positive Mindset: Cultivating Gratitude and Resilience

Living with EDS presents unique challenges, but cultivating a positive mindset, gratitude, and resilience can significantly enhance your quality of life. Here are strategies for fostering a positive outlook and building emotional strength:

1. Practice Gratitude:

Daily gratitude practices, such as keeping a gratitude journal or sharing things you're thankful for with a loved one, can shift your focus from what is challenging to what is positive in your life. This practice can enhance your overall mood and outlook.

2. Mindfulness and Meditation:

Incorporate mindfulness and meditation into your routine to help manage stress and improve emotional resilience. Mindfulness practices can help you stay present and reduce anxiety about the future or regret about the past.

3. Set Realistic Goals:

Set realistic and achievable goals for yourself. Break larger tasks into smaller, manageable steps and celebrate your accomplishments, no matter how small. This approach can boost your confidence and motivation.

4. Connect with Supportive Communities:

Surround yourself with supportive friends, family, and communities. Connecting with others who understand your experiences can provide emotional support and foster a sense of belonging.

5. Engage in Activities You Enjoy:

Pursue hobbies and activities that bring you joy and fulfillment. Whether it's creative arts, reading, nature walks, or volunteering, engaging in enjoyable activities can enhance your overall wellbeing.

6. Develop Coping Strategies:

Identify and develop coping strategies that work for you. These might include deep breathing exercises, progressive muscle relaxation, or engaging in physical activity that suits your abilities.

7. Seek Professional Support:

Don't hesitate to seek professional support from therapists or counselors who can help you navigate the emotional challenges of living with EDS. Cognitive-behavioral therapy (CBT) and other therapeutic approaches can be particularly effective.

8. Celebrate Your Strengths:

Acknowledge and celebrate your strengths and achievements. Remind yourself of your resilience, adaptability, and the unique qualities that make you who you are.

By embracing a positive mindset and cultivating gratitude and resilience, you can navigate the challenges of EDS with greater emotional strength and a sense of hope.

Thriving with EDS involves more than just managing symptoms; it means living a full, rich, and satisfying life despite the challenges. Here are ways to live your best life every day with EDS:

1. Prioritize Self-Care:

Make self-care a non-negotiable part of your daily routine. This includes physical, emotional, and mental health practices that help you feel your best. Regularly assess your needs and adjust your self-care practices accordingly.

2. Build a Support Network:

Surround yourself with a strong support network of family, friends, healthcare providers, and support groups. Having a reliable support system can provide practical assistance, emotional support, and a sense of community.

3. Educate Yourself and Others:

Stay informed about EDS and educate those around you about the condition. Increased awareness can lead to better support and understanding from others, and empower you to advocate effectively for your needs.

4. Adapt Your Environment:

Create a living environment that supports your health and comfort. Use assistive devices and make modifications to your home and workspace to reduce physical strain and enhance accessibility.

5. Engage in Enjoyable Activities:

Make time for activities that you enjoy and that bring you joy. Whether it's a hobby, a creative pursuit, or spending time with loved ones, engaging in pleasurable activities can boost your mood and overall wellbeing.

6. Stay Active:

Incorporate gentle, low-impact exercise into your routine to maintain physical health and mobility. Activities like swimming, yoga, or walking can help you stay active without putting excessive strain on your joints.

7. Plan for Energy Conservation:

Plan your activities and prioritize tasks to conserve your energy. Pacing yourself and taking regular breaks can help you manage fatigue and avoid overexertion.

8. Embrace Flexibility:

Be flexible and adaptable in your approach to daily life. Recognize that some days will be better than others, and adjust your plans and expectations accordingly. Flexibility can help you navigate the unpredictability of EDS.

9. Seek Joy and Fulfillment:

Seek out experiences and opportunities that bring you joy and fulfillment. Focus on what makes you happy and pursue your passions and interests with enthusiasm.

By focusing on self-care, building a strong support network, engaging in enjoyable activities, and embracing flexibility, you can live a full and satisfying life with EDS. Thriving with EDS means finding balance, joy, and fulfillment in your everyday experiences.

CONCLUSION

Living with Ehlers-Danlos Syndrome presents unique challenges, but with the right strategies, support, and mindset, it is possible to live a fulfilling and enriching life. This book has explored various aspects of living with EDS, from understanding the condition and its manifestations to building a supportive community and advocating for yourself. By focusing on self-care, prioritizing your health, and embracing a positive outlook, you can navigate the complexities of EDS and thrive.

Throughout this journey, you've learned about the importance of tailored exercise, proper nutrition, and quality sleep in managing EDS symptoms. You've explored effective pain management strategies and stress-reduction techniques, and discovered the value of open communication and setting boundaries in your relationships. Additionally, you've seen how adapting your environment and finding meaningful work can enhance your quality of life.

Staying informed about the latest research and advancements in EDS treatment, cultivating gratitude and resilience, and seeking joy and fulfillment in your daily activities are key to thriving with EDS. Remember that you are not alone—there is a community of individuals who understand your experiences and can offer support and encouragement.

As you continue your journey, keep in mind that every step you take towards self-care and self-advocacy is a step towards living your best life. Embrace the possibilities, stay hopeful, and celebrate your resilience and strength. With the right tools, support, and mindset, you can live a life filled with purpose, joy, and fulfillment, despite the challenges of EDS.

www.ingramcontent.com/pod-product-compliance
Lightning Source LLC
Chambersburg PA
CBHW071010250726
48653CB00005B/1570